sexcitement

Acknowledgments
My special thanks to all my remarkable friends (they know who they are), some of whom have generously allowed me to use them as models and others who have contributed ideas and shared their personal experiences with such candour.
My thanks also to Sylvie Jones for her wonderfully lively illustrations.

THE *Erotic* Print Society
London 2002

THE *Erotic* Print Society
EPS, 1 Maddox Street
LONDON W1S 2PZ

Tel (UK only): 0800 026 25 24
Fax: +44 (0)20 7437 3528
Email: eros@eps.org
Web: www.eroticprints.org

ISBN : 1-898998-54- X

Printed and bound in Spain by Bookprint, S.L., Barcelona

THE ART OF LOVE

sexcitement

lynn paula russell

pleasures without prejudice

THE *Erotic* Print Society

i *denotes further information to be found at the back of book*

Contents

why sexcitement is important

A CRUCIAL WORD OF CAUTION

Most of the activities described in this book are fun and entirely without risk. Others, on the other hand, are also fun but *could* involve risk unless certain precautions are taken. Good sex need never be – and should never be – dangerous. If a practice or activity is new to you, please don't try to run before you walk. If you're confused or uncertain, seek more advice: there's plenty of it about. Remember *always* to practice 'safe sex' in the sense of using adequate protection against sexually transmitted diseases (STDs) or the HIV virus (which can lead to AIDS) and that includes being aware. But it helps to remember: unless you are having sex with a long-term partner – use a condom!

INTRODUCTION

It is a well-known fact that the moment couples start to form close attachments and live together the greater is the risk that their erotic life will become narrowed down and limited within the safe parameters of the familiar. I once read somewhere that water loses much of its vitality once it has stopped flowing freely and becomes stagnant, and this could be an analogy for what happens to sex, once it stops moving and flowing and settles down into a repetitive, unquestioned routine. Before you know where you are the drive starts to diminish. We might be inclined to deduce that this impulse was not designed for long standing relationships, but do not let this deter you! We are conscious human beings, not animals, and we have imaginations and the ability to grow and change and even transform ourselves.

Young people get married or move in together with every intention of creating a vibrant and passionate erotic life with their beloved, believing that the way they feel now cannot possibly be reduced to the sterile state of affairs they have observed in many of the older generation; but they have a lot to learn! This book aims to provide a few helpful tips for maintaining that much needed lustful sparkle, but mainly it will bring together and explore the fascinating range of erotic variety, including the so-called perversions and taboos, and throw some light into their midst. There is still much fear connected with our sexual behaviour and oddly enough, if offered the choice, most of us would rather go off with a stranger to explore the more deviant aspects of our natures, than share them with the one who is closest to us. This attitude leads to a part of ourselves splitting off and being tucked away in a dark recess, when it could be explored so much more safely and lead to the understanding and deepening of our relationships.

1

fantasy

Adventures
Scenarios
Games

FANTASY

We hear so much about fantasy nowadays. I myself have appeared on a TV documentary in which several women of various ages were invited to talk freely about their private erotic reveries. I remember that we were all quite nervous at the beginning, for we all imagined that our inner life was so much worse than anyone else's. Once we realised that almost every woman there had conjured up similar scenes of gangbangs, incest, naughty adventures with horses or dogs, experiments with members of her own sex, spankings and bondage, we all started to laugh with relief. All these fantasies were quite common. Everyone, without exception, has fantasies and we should not feel ashamed of our own or in any way resentful when we realise that our special partner has secret yearnings too which may or may not include us.

There are two kinds of erotic fantasy: the ones we consciously dream up and spend time polishing and honing for our own arousal, and those others which seem to erupt from nowhere into our minds, perhaps while we masturbate, and develop in directions that may disturb us. The first category represents things that we feel sure we would like if only we could arrange them: our favourite type of man or woman, in a setting and occasion of our choosing, fitting in beautifully to the ideal scene we have composed. However the second category may well consist of childish ingredients, the use of force, even a touch of sheer *dirtiness*. Our civilised selves might heartily despise these thoughts and we do not necessarily even know whether we would enjoy them in reality — if the fantasy features a rape scene we are quite certain we would not.

These are the fantasies we are loath to share with others.

The American artist and sex guru Betty Dodson once said that in our masturbation fantasies we are identifying with all the characters: the men and the women, the submissive and the dominant, the abuser and the abused. I believe she is right and that this notion sheds new light on the subject. What else is the use of fantasy but our need to experience and identify with all the variations of human sexuality, from every point of view? It reveals our need to experience life more fully. Since we are all confined within the boundaries of civilised behaviour and our own morality, not to mention the fact that we have only one body and one gender through which we function, it is obvious that many qualities and situations will remain untasted, particularly those involving dominance and submission. We live in a relatively liberal and caring society today and equality is (quite rightly) the aim, but this means we never get the chance to sample the more extreme situations.

We have no qualms about reading books and watching dramas and documentaries about other people's experiences, but somehow when it comes to sex we can't help feeling a little guilty and prurient if we try to peek in for a quick fix!

But there is more to it than that; I believe that our own unique fantasies, particularly the kind that arise spontaneously and keep preying on our minds, have a personal significance for us. They contain the germ of an idea which, if acknowledged and looked at, could help us to see our own nature more clearly. They are signposts, pointing to an unknown destination, but saying, 'If you go this way you will find something valuable to yourself'. However, the signpost can be highly misleading and I am not for a moment going to suggest that you rush off and try to act out literally every single erotic idea that has ever turned you on.

We need to share our fantasies, and if we can share them with someone who cares for us, so much the better. A much-cherished fantasy can become an empty repetition if it does not move and develop. If repressed it can also become too obsessive and fill us with fear that once let out, this impulse could ramp around wreaking havoc like a lecherous genie released from his bottle.

This book is directed towards those couples who feel they would like to explore a little more widely but are not sure how to start. It is not attempting to tell anyone that they should be dissatisfied with what they do; you must all follow your own inner directives. Trying out new erotic ideas just for the sake of being daring and different is not the object of the exercise.

ADVENTURES

Whenever your life changes direction, or you add something new to it, you are embarking on an adventure, the outcome of which you cannot possibly know. Deciding to share your life with another person is the beginning of a big adventure in itself and part of the excitement of it at the outset is the knowledge that there will be new challenges and unexpected twists and turns along the way because both partners are continuing to grow and develop as individuals; nothing can remain static. This is particularly true of our sex lives. We mustn't be afraid to introduce new directions and keep the spirit of adventure alive.

Sex between two people who care for each other can be particularly invigorating and generate powerful energy for both, as well as a much-needed emotional release when you both have a good orgasm. When we give only part of ourselves to this physical interaction I believe we are imposing limitations on the relationship and diminishing its full potential.

A very small event can trigger off an erotic adventure. Simply breaking a habit and surprising your partner might start it – by not doing what you always do. If you are the one who always waits to be seduced, then try to initiate a lovemaking session yourself. If you always get into a certain position for sex then try something else. Don't be afraid of the spontaneous amusement that might erupt! Vary the clothes you wear, the way you present yourself and don't be afraid to plan surprises. Adventures need a little prompting but they can lead to new discoveries – much more on this in later chapters.

Hidden away deep in my archives I have a small, indistinct Polaroid of myself that I will always keep to remind me of an exciting period in my life. I was living with my partner on the outskirts of London, near a common. We had just acquired a new Polaroid camera (this was more than two decades ago) and it is difficult to explain to those who take for granted the wonders of digital cameras and computer-generated images, exactly how mind-blowingly liberating this simple device was. We could photograph each other in all our intimate glory, and no one at Boots was going to see it and object. To christen this new wonder gadget, my man decided to take me out walking on the common, but stipulated that I was to wear only my knee-length overcoat and a pair of sandals. Feeling excruciatingly vulnerable I complied with his wishes and we went on a photographing spree.

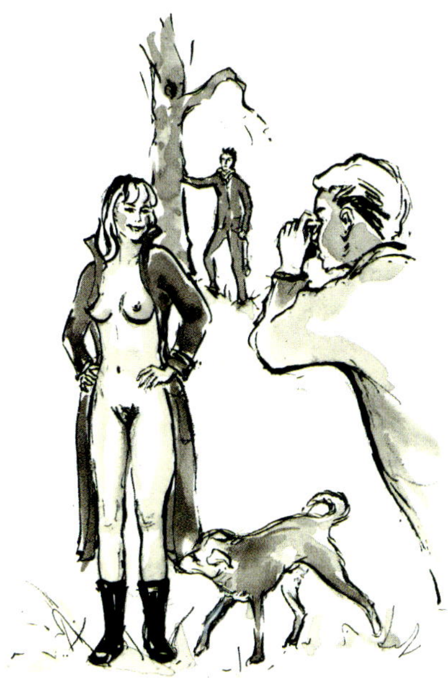

At the end of the day we had a collection of pictures of me standing against the backdrop of the common saucily pulling up my coat to reveal my bare bottom or opening it to give the camera a partial view of my nakedness, while unaware strangers walked their dogs in the background. All very innocent fun. I would never have taken the coat right off because it was not our intention to cause offence, just to amuse each other. My favourite snap is the one we took on the railway station platform. It shows me holding the front of my coat wide open and grinning like a naughty pixie as a group of bored commuters stand disconsolately behind me, looking at their watches as they wait for the delayed train to Liverpool Street.

It was only on the way back that I realised that adventures can have an unexpected twist in their tail: As we made our way along a main road we encountered two old friends who invited us in for a cup of tea. We were about to say yes when I realised that I was not properly dressed for tea parties and since it was a warm day they would have thought it odd if I had sat there insisting on keeping my coat firmly pulled around me. So we made our excuses.

My partner later confessed that he had fought back a wicked desire to accept the invitation, to see what would have happened. Yes, well... I know what would have happened; in those days, absolutely nothing. I was far too self-conscious and conventional to admit my interest in erotic adventures.

SCENARIOS

A scenario is a scene in which partners choose the role they would like to play and improvise around the theme, rather like a theatre workshop — although perhaps that is rather too grand a word for it. None but the best of actors can stay in a role for long without feeling the need to giggle or fall out of character. In this particular context, those two weaknesses are quite permissible and sometimes even add to the enjoyment. It is always a game after all, and supposed to release you, not make you feel you must give a skilled performance. Whether you decide to play the part of the whore, the gigolo, the innocent girl or boy losing their virginity, the lady of the manor misbehaving with the stable boy, or the headmaster chastising the naughty schoolgirl, it is the emotional element that counts, not the standard of acting or attention to costume. If anything, the *more* you try in that department, the more absurd it may become. All you need is to agree on the rules and off you go.

This form of amateur dramatics may not appeal to everyone. I know many who say that sexual happenings should be left to spontaneous chance but I don't believe that that is always a good idea. Knowing in advance that something is about to happen allows you the delicious pleasure of anticipation while you prepare yourself for what lies ahead. Leaving too much to chance can mean that nothing happens at all! Now here I must point out that women, on the whole, do not seem to favour the idea of thinking ahead and planning a scenario in every minute detail as much as men do, especially if it is done too rigidly. However, if you are one of those people who is aroused by being told what is to be done to you then there can be days of teasing and build-up and the imagination can run riot.

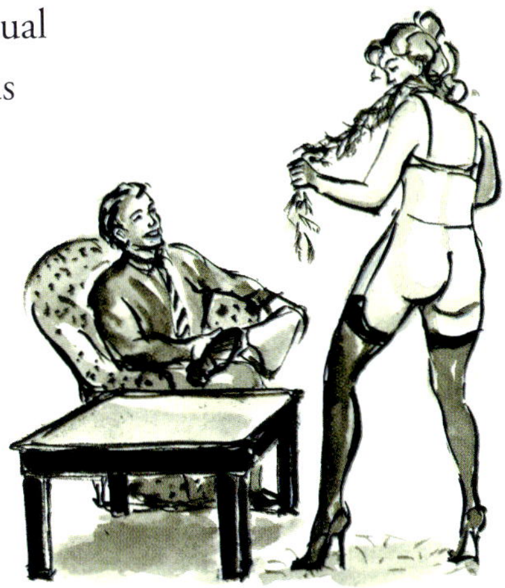

Playing the Whore

A good idea is to have a loose framework, where one of you knows the direction you are heading in, but not every single move that will be made.

For this to work it is advisable for one of you to be in control and this leads us on to the need for *trust* – an important subject I'll be examining in more depth later.

My partner and I used to have the occasional 'submission' day. This meant that for twelve hours or so one of us would be in charge of the other and could command them to do our bidding. These special days were a wonderful opportunity for trying out ideas but also showed up unexpected weaknesses. For instance, on the days when I was in charge, so ingrained was my inhibition about asking for sensual pleasures that I often failed to come up with anything to my advantage! Instead, all my secret female resentments towards men welled up to the surface, and I frittered away my three wishes on futile attempts to get him to strip naked and do the housework!

His days in charge were much more successful, for in me he discovered that behind the moody, stubborn exterior lay a natural tendency for me to be submissive and this became the starting point for new experiences.

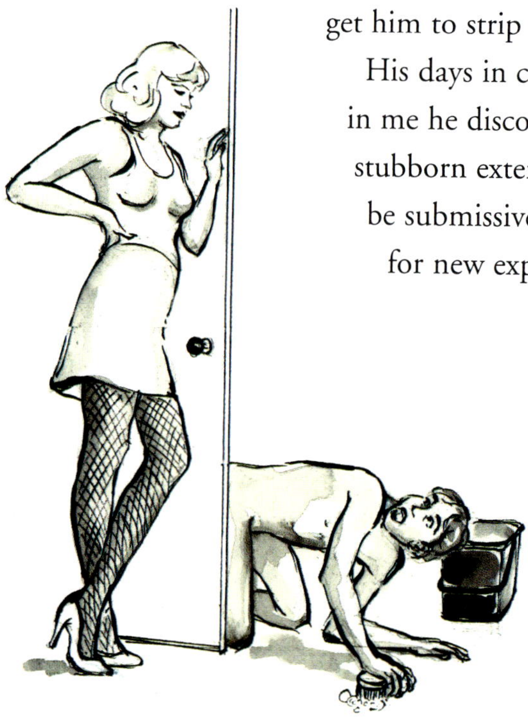

GAMES

Games, and acting out scenarios, may *not* suggest anything very arousing or erotic to those shy people who used to cringe with embarrassment at children's birthday parties whenever the inevitable musical chairs or charades was suggested. I would be the first to agree that infantile games can be distinctly off-putting when they are used to jolly along an otherwise unpromising collection of people, especially if the activities concerned are designed to bring people's bodies naughtily in contact, at the same time as forbidding anything really sexual to develop.

Simply forget all those pathetic attempts at human contact and false hilarity and think more of the kind of games that can help break the ice by using *chance* to dictate the outcome; think of those which can produce an atmosphere enabling people to get in touch with their childlike selves, rather than their gross or infantile selves.

Any game that uses dice can be excellent when adapted for erotic purposes. Just the dice itself, if used with carefully considered options can have amazing results — but more about that later. You can also use any sort of quiz or simple card game framework, adding in your own choice of erotic rewards and punishments.

I can remember a rare evening of unplanned delights. It was one of those times when the right combination of people just happened to come together. We weren't sure what to do with the evening until a close friend of mine, who has a wicked imagination, suggested we try out a special board game I had just been given as a birthday present. It appeared to be a sort of Monopoly with sexy forfeits, but when my friend went through these so-called forfeits she threw most of them out in disgust and declared that she could think of some far better ones; instead of polite little punishments and rewards she wrote some of her own which were not for the faint-hearted.

When the game got underway we were all (apart from my friend) experiencing understandable trepidation; I felt concerned that one of the party in particular might become sullen and intractable if challenged too far, but I needn't have worried, for this is where the die comes in handy and decides what is best for the occasion. It decided, in its wisdom, that the awkward new member of our circle was the one to take off all his kit first, and much to my astonishment, he did it readily and revelled in his nudity (it was obvious that he had been dying to show off his beautiful physique). On the other hand I, who had been quite happy to take my clothes off if my forfeits had dictated, found instead that I was obliged to put extra clothes on as the evening progressed. But I did earn more than my fair share of spankings, mainly dished out by a lady I hardly knew, who had never done such a thing before. Then I got the chance to deliver a short sharp whacking with a leather belt, to her husband of all people. I wonder if that started a new trend for them. We ended the evening with genuine laughter and hugs all round.

Of course, playing games with several friends may not be the kind of thing you are ready for; it does depend on knowing people rather well and feeling comfortable with them.

2

role play

Learning to Trust
Finding the Child in Yourself
Exploring the Power Dynamics
Masochism and Sadism
Punishments
A Touch of Pain as Stimulation
Light Bondage
Fetish and Fashion

LEARNING TO TRUST

I'd like to go back to the idea of the actors' workshop now. I can remember, during my early days in the theatre, having to attend these nightmarish activities and always curling up in anguish inside in case I should dry up and have nothing to say or worse still, be asked to participate in an improvisation which would take me beyond the point that my inhibitions permitted. This is probably the way most of us feel as we embark on something completely new. When the inhibitions go and trust is built up, however, the idea of the improvisation is much less daunting and becomes enormous fun.

I would say that you are not able to be a really good husband or wife until you are at least aware of all the baggage you have brought with you into the relationship. We would probably have been horrified in our youth if we had realised just how many distortions and misapprehensions we had grown up with regarding the opposite sex. If it were not for sexual attraction it is quite likely that we wouldn't be bothered with them at all.

Any relationship of erotic love is likely to be emotionally unstable from time to time, at least to start with; the more passionate it is, the more volatile the emotions. Even under the surface of apparent love there can lurk its complete opposite. Building up trust between a man and a woman needs time and a lot of care, but it is well worth the effort. Without trust there can be little real exploration of new lovemaking techniques, and entering into scenes involving dominance and submission could be a very risky business indeed.

If you need to explore how far you want to go and build up the trust between you and your partner, I would suggest a little experimentation by using a blindfold; if one of you is made to feel exposed and vulnerable you will start to be aware of your dependency upon the other. It can be very exciting for your lover not to know exactly what is to be done to them.

Ask your partner to strip completely naked and then put the blindfold on them, making sure that all the light has been shut out. Next, get them to relax on the bed and make them promise that they will not caress themselves or try to take off the blindfold. Leave the room and let them lie where they are in silent anticipation for as long as you like. Go and look for some items which will produce an array of different sensations: for example, oil to massage them, some ice cubes to give them a rude awakening, a soft feather or paint brush to stroke them in sensitive places, maybe a heated spoon to press fleetingly to a nipple (be careful here). Try running the ice cubes down their body, or into their crevices and then follow that swiftly with the warmth of your breath on the same area of skin. Experiment with how far a caressing sensation can go before it starts to become the beginnings of a pain. Extremely soft suede thongs are excellent for this as they can be trailed enticingly between the legs and over the stomach and then flapped and flicked to produce a stimulating sting. A full-blown thwack should not be tried unexpectedly, as that is hardly likely to increase a person's trust and will only make them tense and nervous. It is the amount you restrain yourself and tune in to them which will help build the acceptance and full trust between you.

The most important aspect of this is that both parties know how the sensations feel, both to administer and receive: this will help them to know the effect of what they are doing to their partner.

To feel even more vulnerable and dependent, try this exercise outdoors. If you have a suitable park without too many dog walkers, go out on a warm night and try entrusting yourself to your partner, or the other way round. When you have reached a sheltered spot, let him/her blindfold you and lead you around (when I did this I felt sure I was about to be led

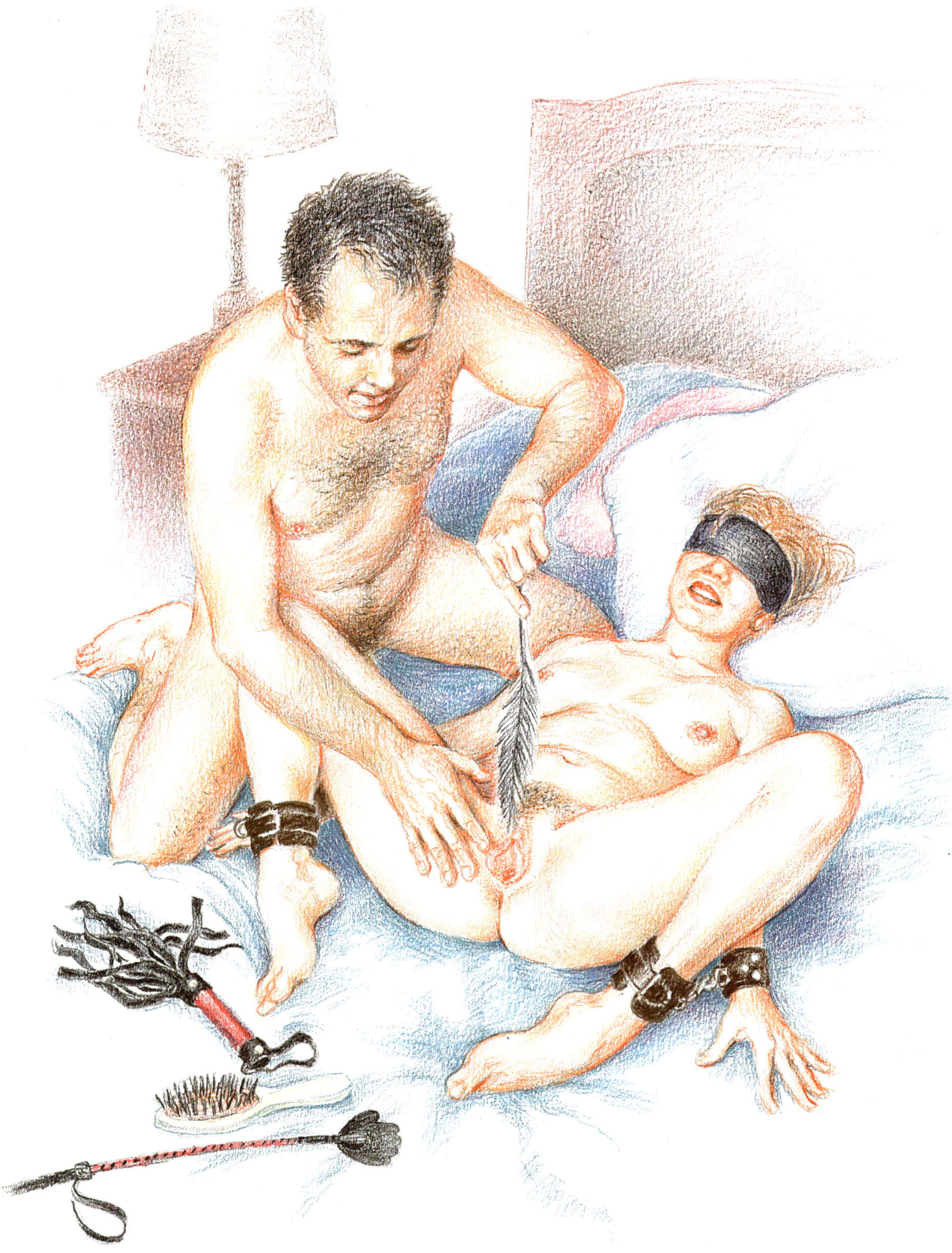

Exploring Sensations

into the nearest thorn bush) then let yourself be settled on a grassy spot chosen by the sighted one, and lie back. Your partner will then uncover you as much as possible (easier to accomplish with a women wearing a skirt than with a man zipped up in trousers) and leave you blindfolded and exposed to contemplate the sounds and perfumes of the night. This can be an exquisite experience, but one in which you will need all the trust you can muster. Every crackle in the undergrowth will set your nerves tingling and the darkness and strangeness will lead you to think that you have been staked out for a passing rapist or wild animal — the fact that your lover is standing not more than three yards away, watching over you, will make no difference whatsoever. Then comes the moment when you hear him/her approaching and feel a gentle finger caressing between your legs or a wet tongue licking up your thigh (*now* you can see why I stipulated that there should be no dog walkers or dogs in the vicinity), and the memory of that experience will stay with you forever.

You can go on to try the blindfold routine at home adding some light bondage. Prepare your partner by bending their legs back over their tummy and tie their ankles to their wrists with a soft scarf or cuffs, if you have them. This keeps the arms out of the way and makes sure that the legs stay put in a most revealing position. Another way to tie them is on all fours, with the wrists again tied to the ankles; this will make sure they are presented in one of the most exposed positions imaginable.

Talking of exposing, it might be helpful to be aware at this stage that for some people, because they have been told they are dirty or shameful, certain parts of the body will be closed off and not necessarily considered to be erogenous. I am thinking particularly of the area between the buttocks, around the anus. If you try to stroke them here they will automatically clench their cheeks, and become tense. This is a good time to try and work on this supersensitive area, reassuring your partner that every inch of them is pleasing to you, and potentially the source of great sensual enjoyment to them. Their buttocks must be gently coaxed apart so that their anus and perineum can be stroked lovingly with a feather and teased with your tongue.

An important point to be kept in mind is that as long as there is muscular tension, caused by fear or resentment, it will be impossible to enter completely into the spirit of erotic discovery. What's more, any experiments involving pain as a form of stimulation will probably be a dismal failure if your body is stiff and tense. Even the most gentle of spanking play can become painful and the opposite of arousing if the recipient does not accept what is being done, or run with it and allow it to flow through them.

FINDING THE CHILD IN YOURSELF

If a human being is anything like a tree trunk, adding ring upon ring of growth and new experience as the years go by, then it stands to reason that the central nucleus of childhood remains the oldest part of any individual. Those early layers have been there since the beginning and are always present when the more mature outer persona crumbles through tiredness or stress.

Exactly when a young person first starts to become aware of sex remains a mystery. The actual mechanics of it may be vague to the young mind until quite near puberty, but the awareness of gender and powerplay is there at an early age, as well as the knowledge that certain areas of the body are more 'rude' than others and liable to cause giggling and excitement when shown or talked about.

It is quite laughable that we lump all sex films and magazines in a category called 'adult' entertainment. I mean – sitting around avidly discussing the ideas of Plato and Socrates and the development of Western philosophy is an *adult* pursuit. Watching King Lear at the National is an *adult* entertainment. But what strikes me as being in a different category altogether is lying back gasping as someone's tongue tickles your clitoris, or watching someone suck lustily on a shiny pink knob as if it were a lollypop.

Finding the child in you means getting in touch with that child-like innocence, with the side of yourself that can giggle at the absurdity of our physical habits, at the same time as thoroughly enjoying them. It means being completely non-judgmental and reacting spontaneously as a child would. One of the biggest discoveries of my life was to realise that sex, in itself, as a natural appetite, when you are fully involved of your own free will, is one of the most innocent of impulses. It only becomes dark and sordid when exploitation or manipulation creeps in.

So, don't be afraid to be plain childish together; you've nothing to hide with the person who loves you. Probably one of the most comforting ways to recover from stress and anxiety is to return briefly to a world unencumbered by the awareness of consequences, where responsibility was only something that others had towards us. Our first taste of this was at our mother's breast, and this simple interaction can also be sexily reassuring to an adult. To be cradled by your partner/lover/surrogate mother as she presents her nipple to you for nuzzling and suckling can help to shut out all woes. You can bury your face in her breasts and drink deep of the perfume of her skin. I know that some go further than the simulated drinking and grab the opportunity for a taste of mother's milk itself when their wives *are* actually breast-feeding, but this is rather more difficult to arrange!

For women, sitting snuggled on a male lap can have the same effect (unless, of course, you had an unfortunate experience on the lap of a

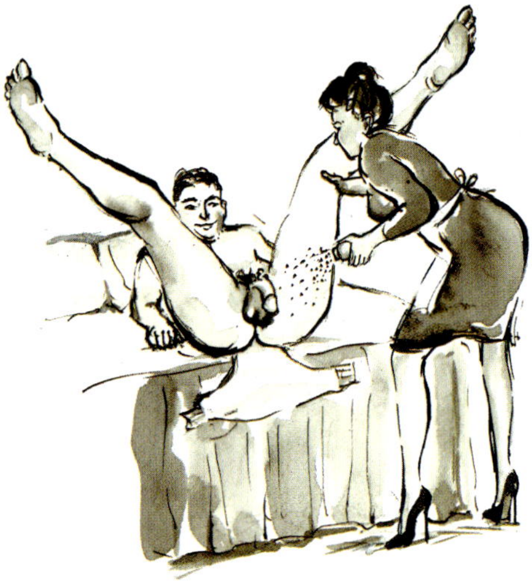

Adult Nappy Changing

distant male relative when you were in your Shirley Temple years!).

I know that some people like to go the whole hog: wearing plastic knickers, wetting themselves, having their nappies changed and receiving generous talcum powdering to their overdeveloped baby's buttocks, before being placed in their playpens. All I can say here is this: go ahead and try it if you feel so inclined. If these activities help to build up trust and intimacy between you and your partner then that's all that need concern you.

A good place for childish pursuits is in the bathroom. I always feel immediately transported back to my choldhood when someone washes me in the bath with a soapy sponge, as my mother used to do (floating ducks optional). You step out of the water, all dripping and steaming, to be enveloped in a huge bath towel and every inch of you is gently patted dry (the patting can be a lot more thorough with your man than with your dear mamma). For anyone who feels a strong desire to play up, here is a good moment. There is nothing like the feeling of a playful hand spanking a very naughty bottom when your body is gorgeously warm and glistening with moisture! The blood is very near the surface of the skin and this makes the spanking more stimulating than painful. For the repeat offenders I really think that a good wooden bath brush should be kept handy to teach them to behave themselves! To round off this experience carry the chastened woman in your arms into the bedchamber.

To get yourself in the mood for further nostalgic reveries, you can try getting hold of the kind of undies that bring back memories of the younger you. Mainly it is female apparel I am thinking of here, since I don't believe that young girls fantasised much about what young boys were wearing under their shorts. I am quite certain, though, that most young boys had an obsessive interest in the kind of garments that covered the lower regions of their female friends. I only have to see those pairs of large navy or white cotton knickers and I am immediately transported back to the days of PE lessons, playing 'hospitals' with the boys next door and sometimes 'Truth or Dare' in our garden shed. In our very young teens, we girls used to worry a great deal about the secret parts of our bodies being seen. To have a towel unexpectedly fall down while you were changing out of your swimming costume on the beach was an excruciating indignity never to be lived down, and it is exactly this super-sensitivity (and accompanying excitement) that we lose as we get more used to taking our clothes off in front of members of the opposite sex. All the same, the intensity of feeling associated with childhood is still there inside us, just waiting to be released.

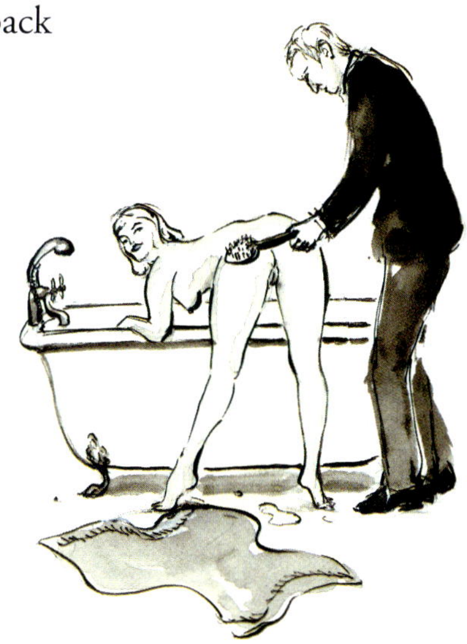

Spanking With the Bath Brush

Having the right clothes for the part does help you get into character. A woman, at whatever age, is bound to feel foolishly young when dressed in a short pleated skirt, white blouse, ankle socks and hair in bunches, or a man in short trousers and schoolboy cap. Yes, we might look silly to an outside eye, especially if we happen to be over fifty, but who cares? These are our own *private* fantasies and it is no one's business but ours. It may not be a popular subject these days but we all know that some women love to be put over their man's knee and soundly spanked; it reminds them of something intensely reassuring, that someone cares enough to discipline them. However, don't make the mistake of assuming that *all* women will respond to this sort of treatment – for some it may bring back unwelcome memories that should be left alone.

For some men, bending over for an application of the slipper or ruler to their bare bottoms by a school mistress (you) can be intensely exciting, but you must both take it seriously enough. The lecture the malcontent receives before the punishment must be delivered with confidence and the whacking must be firm and real enough to satisfy. The role-playing from the 'pupil' may include a quavering little voice, blushing cheeks and eyes cast down in shame at the floor, but follow it through and the barriers will come down. I've known many who say that these games are cathartic, as well as being highly arousing.

To conclude this section I'd just like to say that indulging the child in yourself can be wonderfully liberating to start with but you must be careful that the childish ego does not try to take you over. Children do love repeating the same exercises time and again and if you let this happen to you, your fantasy life could get into some pretty tiresome habit patterns.

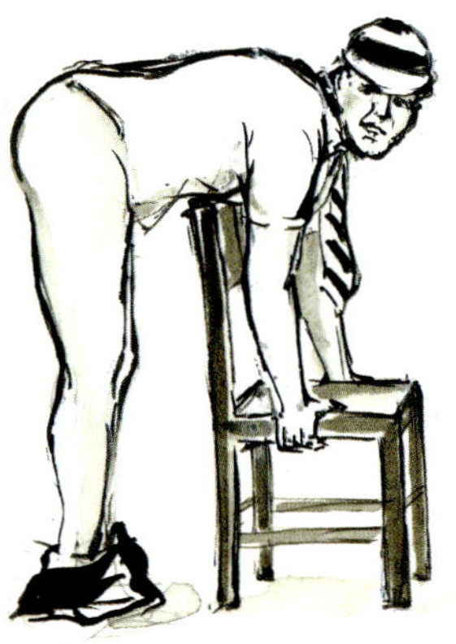

Bending Over for the Head Mistress

EXPLORING THE POWER DYNAMIC: DOMINANCE AND SUBMISSION

I have often wondered why most of our private

erotic fantasies contain such a strong element of power play. Is this the ingredient that creates the electricity of sex? Making love and respecting another's wishes is what we genuinely work towards in our conscious life, but when it comes to fantasy we often go to great lengths to invent situations in which we can manoeuvre someone else to do our bidding. Few of us usually enjoy straightforward forcing – that's just crude, and a sign of weakness – but many of us do love, in fantasy, a good excuse for exploiting a situation outrageously. Being able to command another is a very heady experience. Equally, there are those who can't face their own appetites and shrink from initiating anything for themselves, and they rejoice in being led on by another and forced to do all those things they secretly want to do but never dared ask for.

Here is our chance to bring out some of those secret desires but I know from talking to many couples that it is not always easy to start along this route. Who is willing to go first and be honest? If your relationship is based on equality, how do you suddenly take the plunge and allow your partner to take charge of you? And if there are already resentments and power struggles bubbling under the surface it becomes doubly difficult.

We don't always know what we really want to do until we have tried it. I knew someone once who enjoyed looking at images of women bending over to be spanked, and fantasised no end about it. When he finally got his dream and a flesh and blood woman lay expectantly across his lap, he was baffled to find that it left him cold: he hadn't realised that all along he had been identifying with the 'victim'!

I remember a woman who spent much of her time putting down her husband in front of other people; I often thought that given her head she would become the quintessential snarling dominatrix, but now I realise that this wasn't necessarily so: she was probably impatient with her husband because he wasn't firm enough with her. He might have been surprised to see how meekly she would have responded to him if only he had found the right way to deal with her.

To break the deadlock of starting, I advise giving the dice a try. By allowing the dice to make a decision, you avoid either one of you being held responsible for the choices that are made. So, the first move is for both of you to agree to abide by the dice's decision. Then you choose the options, and this is the fascinating part. On an evening or day when you have time to yourselves, using only the one six-sided die to start with, think of six different erotic activities (three each) that you would like to do or have done to you. Two of them can be fairly usual, but one of them must be a shot in the dark, a dare if you like. Let's see, you could put down:

Her –

1. He gives me cunnilingus
2. I tie his arms to the bed and we fuck with me on top
3. I tie him to the bed and whack him with my hairbrush

Him –

4. She gives me a blow job
5. I fuck her in any position I choose
6. She dresses in her sexiest undies, does a strip tease for me and then masturbates so that I can watch

Of course, the options will depend on what is a challenge to you personally; some couples might find any one of the above a challenge, while others might find all of them completely acceptable, or even commonplace. If you are one of the latter, then a lot more imagination is called for. Throw the die only once and whatever comes up you must do it, without argument or conditions.

If number three comes up then throw two dice to see how many strokes should be given. Of course, if this is the first time either of you have experimented with implements, do take it gently to start with (see next section).

Probably the most difficult option for me would be number six, and this, incidentally, was the one request that 'O' (Pauline Réage's heroine in *The Story of O*) found impossible to carry out. It may sound easy, but revealing your own private masturbation methods can be extremely challenging, not to mention the preliminary strip act!

When one of your own options comes up it will be interesting to note the different feelings: for example, if it is 'He gives me cunnilingus' the female partner will feel that at last, here is her chance to make him do it as she wants it done and for as long a time as she wants it, as opposed to the more usual situation where she might feel that it's awfully nice of him to take the trouble and she ought to be a bit grateful, and if she takes a long time to reach orgasm his poor tongue might get strained... Girls – put all this out of your heads; if the die has selected one of your options, it means you have been given full permission to lie back and enjoy. Grab the opportunity and don't be bashful!

A direction will soon emerge from these experiments, for it is often those spontaneous, slightly barmy suggestions – the ones that make you feel nervous and excited at the same time – which the die insists on selecting! How far you want to go into full-blown dominance and submission will unfold gradually. Once the dice have played their part and helped you over the first hurdles, it's time to make up your own mind what happens next.

Start to flesh out the scenarios and think of the best way to get your partner to fulfil your wishes. Your voice must be firm and confident, no need to shout or push them around. There are better ways to command

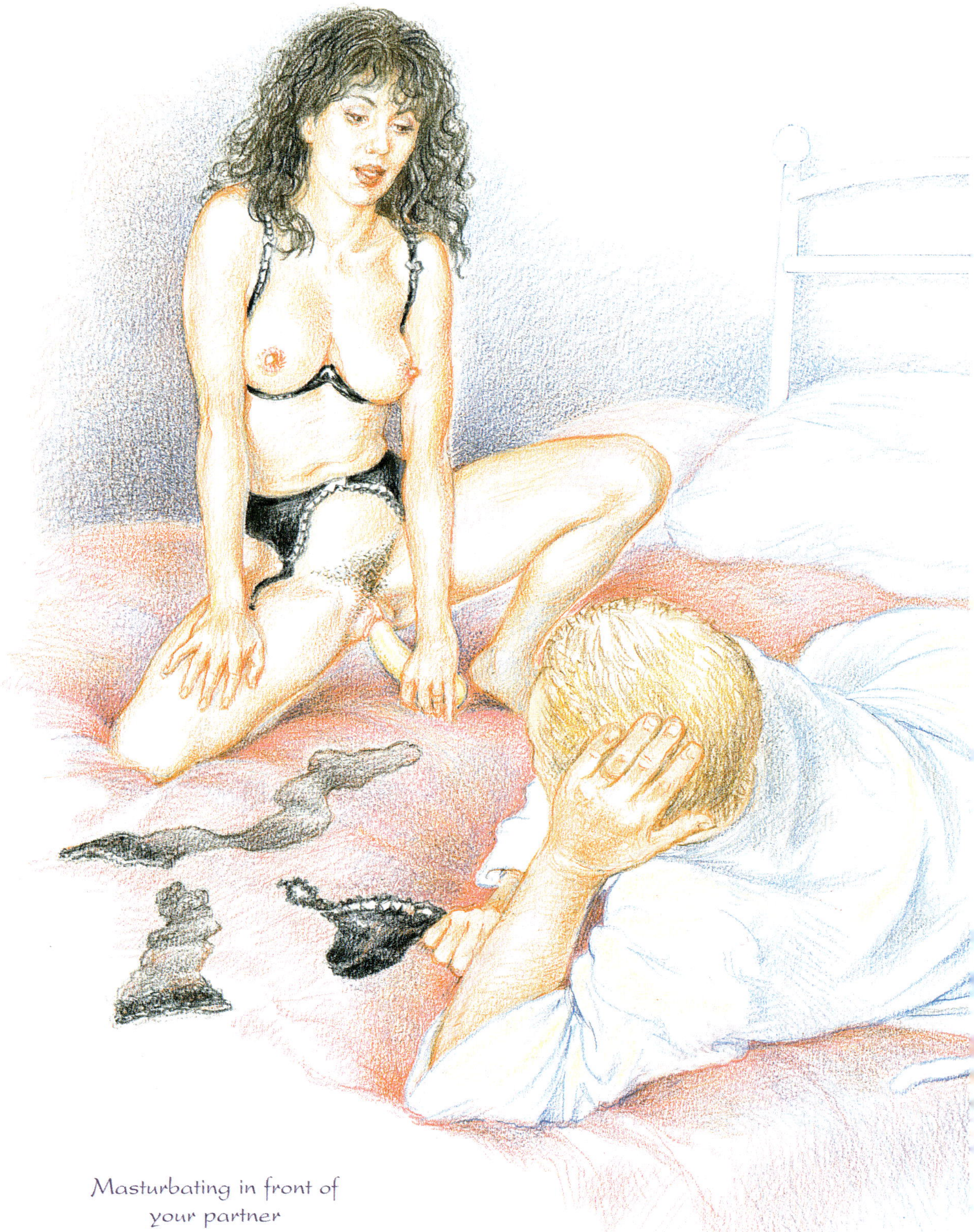

Masturbating in front of
your partner

obedience than that, and once you get a feeling for it you will think of embellishments. There is a kind of discipline which demands no extraneous chatter or giggling and builds towards a higher concentration of intensity. Never give your partner a vague request like, 'Lick me… down there', or worse still, chicken out of saying anything by pushing his head hopefully in a downward direction. That simply will not do! If you want your man to run his tongue delicately around the lips of your cunt or tickle your clitoris, then you must try to say this clearly, and you must make sure he does exactly what you wish and, most important, if you tell him to stop, he must obey immediately, even if he has only just begun to get into his stride.

There are two kinds of challenges for the one who elects to be dominant: getting the reticent person to open up more and secondly, getting the over-enthusiastic, domineering person under control! The former situation may apply more often to men and require great patience, while the latter applies more often to women, for whom dominating means using a strong will to keep under control a more powerful and unruly beast than themselves, as a rider controls an excitable horse!

This exercise will be good for you if you are one of those people who finds talking about sexual matters brings on an attack of the stutters. If you are not accustomed to demanding what you want it will be devilishly difficult at first but very good practice. All those secretive souls who start a sex session hoping that their partner will give them what they want by some means of telepathy will have to work harder than anyone else, but there should be some revelations

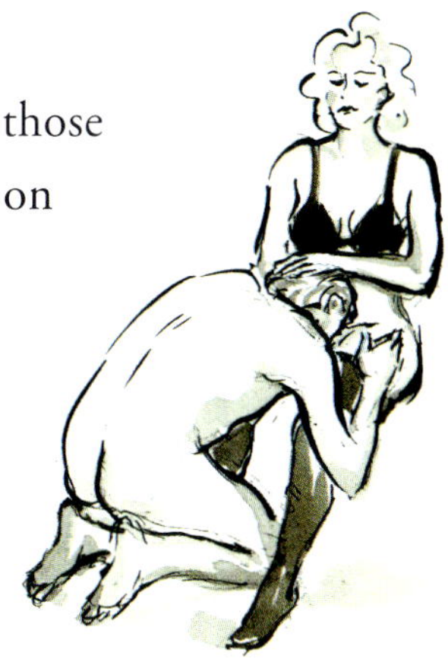

Power Dynamics

along the way. You will know a lot more about what really works for one another.

I know that there are lots of different kinds of 'acts' that couples like to try out, involving a sort of worship at one end of the spectrum, to the use of humiliation and insults at the other. All these elements can come into our minds once we give ourselves permission, but personally I would not encourage the use of insults and humiliation in the treatment of anyone, as this can stir up negativity and resentment. Sooner or later, however, there will be the need for some people to explore the use of pain and punishment, as this seems to be a vital ingredient which crops up naturally in many popular fantasies. Lots of us adore being naughty and would be most disappointed if it did not lead to a good spanking. In fact there are those who maintain that it is these erotic chastisements that act as a valuable outlet for emotional detritus, helping to keep their relationship on an even keel.

MASOCHISM AND SADISM

It is an interesting point that a lot of us have no idea whether we are either masochists or sadists. We assume that just because we don't hurt anyone physically or enjoy pain, that we know nothing of these qualities, when in reality we may be hurting people in other ways by cruelly putting them down in conversations, or alternatively, unconsciously constructing situations in which we can be the one to suffer and make everyone else feel guilty! I only mention that because I used to do the latter.

Male masochism is well described in the works of Leopold von Sacher Masoch who placed the strong dominant female at the centre of his erotic world and revelled in the various harsh cruelties she meted out; the female variety is best shown in Pauline Réage's *The Story of O*. Both contain elements of pseudo-religious desire to worship some facet of the mistress or master and allow them to become the raison d'être of the slave's existence. In other words it is not the pain in itself that is the arousing factor, but the circumstances and relationship between the two people concerned which is built up in a subtle interplay so that the onlooker cannot be sure who is the true driving force.

There is a less complicated way of looking at this subject, though; a certain kind of pain can be seen simply as a stimulus. When combined with the right sort of emotional role-play it can be particularly effective, but for some it can still work perfectly well without those trappings. I once heard a fascinating interview on Radio 4 with an experienced professional dominatrix who pointed out very clearly that she had three different kinds of client: those who came to her to act out scenes (maybe unresolved emotional episodes from their past), those who simply wanted the gratification of skilfully applied pain, and thirdly, those who enjoyed a particular fetish. Most people who are tempted to experiment in this area will probably find that all three of these aspects can combine together, but one will probably turn out to predominate.

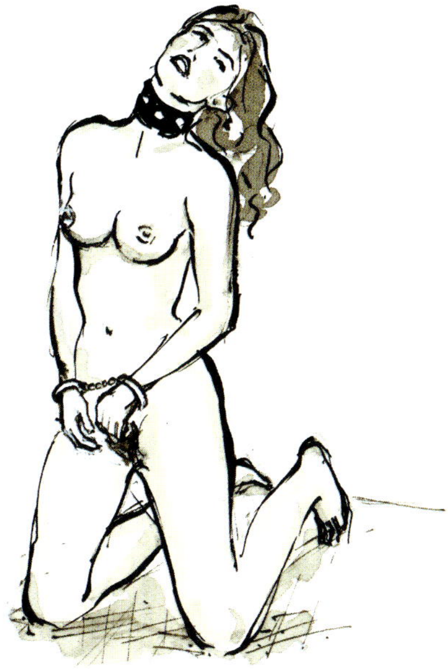

Female Submission

If we take a look at sadism by studying its founder, the wicked Marquis, we will be none the wiser. He was not a good advertisement for what we are discussing here for he was endlessly insisting that people were either totally of one persuasion or the other (we will never know if he actually believed it), whereas, in reality, it makes more sense to assume that we all have a bit of both. Of the two drives, the desire to inflict pain on others is slightly easier to understand than its opposite, but a lot harder to accept in oneself.

To further confuse the issue, those with sadistic tendencies do not necessarily have dominant personalities and masochists are not automatically submissive. Thus you can have a highly forceful individual who happens to enjoy bending over like a schoolboy to receive a caning because it turns him on, but doesn't want the lecturing and put-downs that frequently accompany that type of scenario. Equally, there is the meek and quiet person who likes to punish people by encouraging them to walk into painful situations of their own volition or loves to watch others carry out a punishment.

Most of us, at first, wouldn't dream of classifying pain as an exciting stimulus; we associate it more with toothache or the agony of stubbing a toe – not pleasant at all, although you must admit that as far as the second example is concerned, at least you do feel woken up by this sudden outburst in the nerve endings, and because of it there is a discharge of energy (causing you to leap around and say, 'Oh shit!' or something).

There are different ways of using this stimulus; a rhythmic build up with hand or implement which gradually warms up the skin until you feel you can take more, or the shor, sharp tweak of a nipple or prick with a pin. In the first case some people say that once you get into the general flow there is a breaking down of emotional barriers and a heightening of arousal, which is probably why the Victorians loved flagellation so much – they must have had strong emotional blocks to overcome in order to relax their 'stiff upper lip' sufficiently to have a straightforward fuck. But on the other hand, because chastisement of the buttocks frequently caused excitement in both the punished and the punisher, it was a very moot point as to whether corporal punishment actually worked as a deterrent at all! This is not to say that punishments were always pleasurable – far from it.

Most people who have entered into sexual activities involving pain will tell you that it is hardly ever the pain itself that delights them; it is the after-effect – the warm glow of the buttocks spreading to the genitals, the heightened adrenalin rush and the emotional relief. It is all very personal and everyone reacts differently; our nerves give us varying sensations according to how we feel, the temperature of the room we are in and, a vital point, how far we have consented to and accept what is being done.

Is there any such thing as a true masochist? Well, let's just say that there are many people who are able to translate pain into a sort of pleasure (which does not mean that they feel pain *as* pleasure) and if we take that a little further, one can begin to see sadists as those who enjoy 'pleasuring' masochists, but I wouldn't rely on that as a general definition. *Real* sadists will refuse to apply the whip if they know you are going to enjoy it. They will look around for something else that you don't like!

PUNISHMENTS

If you are not the sort of person who can envisage just getting on and spanking your partner's bottom for no better reason than that you both enjoy it, then you will prefer to set up a situation and assume a special chastising personality. I have to be honest here and tell you that I have not met many married couples or long-term partners who regularly go in for acting out punishment scenarios, except of the most light-hearted variety, for the idea of half an hour of fault-finding and castigation as a preamble to a fun spanking doesn't always sit well with the domestic

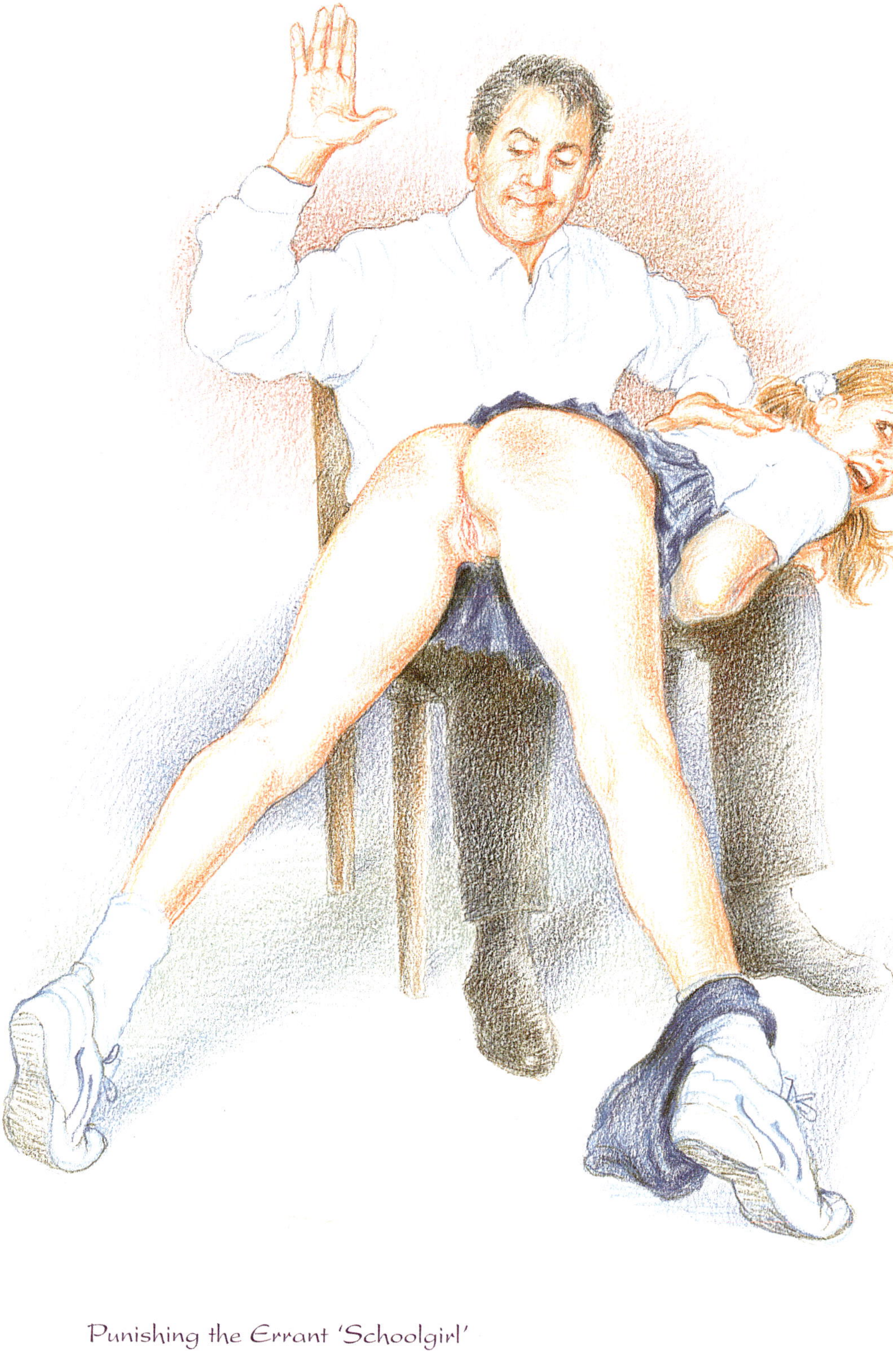

Punishing the Errant 'Schoolgirl'

atmosphere. However I have come across a few couples who are notable exceptions to this.

The thought of being spanked regularly by my husband because I had spent too much money or been cheeky would smack too much of an odious Victorian past; it would be so off-putting that I do not believe it could place me in an erotic frame of mind. But that's just me and each couple must find the fantasy that most excites them, for it is this erotic excitement that puts a completely different complexion on the whole business. To be on the safe side, it is probably better to keep one's erotic peccadilloes separate from the real misdemeanours that could cause the flare-up of unpleasant emotions.

Punishments throughout history have usually been delivered on the back or the buttocks, and for obvious reasons the lovely, fleshy globes of the bottom are a favourite focus of attention for most people who feel attracted to this fantasy.

Every first experience will be sparked off in a different way, and it is preferable if there is enthusiasm and spontaneity from you and your partner. Always look out for signs and try to read them correctly. A woman or man who secretly craves a sound spanking will often try to provoke it by playing up in a childish way and even poking their bottom out invitingly. Sometimes they may do this without even being aware of it. It is up to you to grab the opportunity by playing up to their game. From the other point of view, if your man keeps dropping phrases into the conversation like, 'You deserve a spanked bottom for that!', or 'I have a good mind to warm your arse!', it is very unlikely that he says this purely in jest. Whenever someone brings up certain things time and time again it usually means they have that certain something very much on their mind. There are those who always notice a shapely bottom first, before any other attribute, and they are the ones

closely associated with discipline and chastisement should produce such an array of entertainments – even humour – in those who get involved in it. Going back to the days of childhood, the idea of bending over and showing your bare bottom to the world was an exquisite joke in itself.

The classic spanking position, of course, is over the knee: this brings the spanker and the spanked into close contact. If you are lying over your man's lap it will immediately be made known to you if the treatment he is giving you has had a physical effect on him, for don't forget that he is getting a fine close-up view of your arse cheeks and pussy lips, whereas you are stuck with a close-up of the carpet! This means that there is nothing to divert you from the intense sensations you are experiencing.

Always remember that when the flesh is cold, it registers pain much more acutely, so start any spanking by warming up the area. This means increasing the harshness of the slaps gradually and pausing often to stroke and massage the buttocks to see how they are coming along. Some people may like to start the warm-up over the knickers/boxers and then slowly pull them off, for the removal of underwear prior to a spanking can be an important part of the arousal and should not be rushed. Everybody has a different pain threshold and some skin types will turn red very quickly, others not at all but this doesn't necessarily mean that a more powerful wallop is called for. You can get the strength just right if you experiment with the shape of your hand and the angle at which you bring it down. You will be more effective if your hand is slightly cupped. I think if you are going to try this you might as well do it with gusto; a half-hearted slap is no use to anyone!

There are those who enjoy making no end of a din when they are in the throws of a spanking and there are those who remain as silent as a statue, regardless of what they are feeling. I would say that a little bit of gasping and squealing is fun, whether it is caused by real suffering or just because you enjoy making a rumpus! At any rate you will be giving your chastiser some feedback. He/she does need something to go on. Rapport between the two of you is essential.

USING IMPLEMENTS

Now perhaps you are considering going further and wish to try some implements. This is where we need to be much more careful, for the amount of pain you can inflict on your partner is increased tenfold, particularly with long, thin implements which whizz round in an arc, building up extra speed in the tip so that it lands with more force than you realise. Always practise on an inanimate target – like a cushion – before you use anything on living flesh, for each varying implement requires a different skill. It is also a good idea to make a rule that you never use any implement on a person unless you have thoroughly tested it on yourself!

I believe that if erotic CP is for you, then you will recognise your favourite implement when it comes along. Mine was the slender leather riding crop and I formed an attachment to this partly because it can be an elegant shape in itself (and I love the smell of leather), and partly because it conjured up images of shapely women in tight riding breeches mounted on handsome steeds. The whip is applied to the horse's rump to make him gallop and excel himself, and this, I fancied, would be the effect on me. Mainly I was not disappointed, but I must warn you that this is not a good implement to use at the outset – it can strike with a pain like white-hot fire. A far better way to find your level is to search around the house and select implements from your ordinary household objects. You will find that they fall into two main categories: soft leather items and hard wooden or plastic ones.

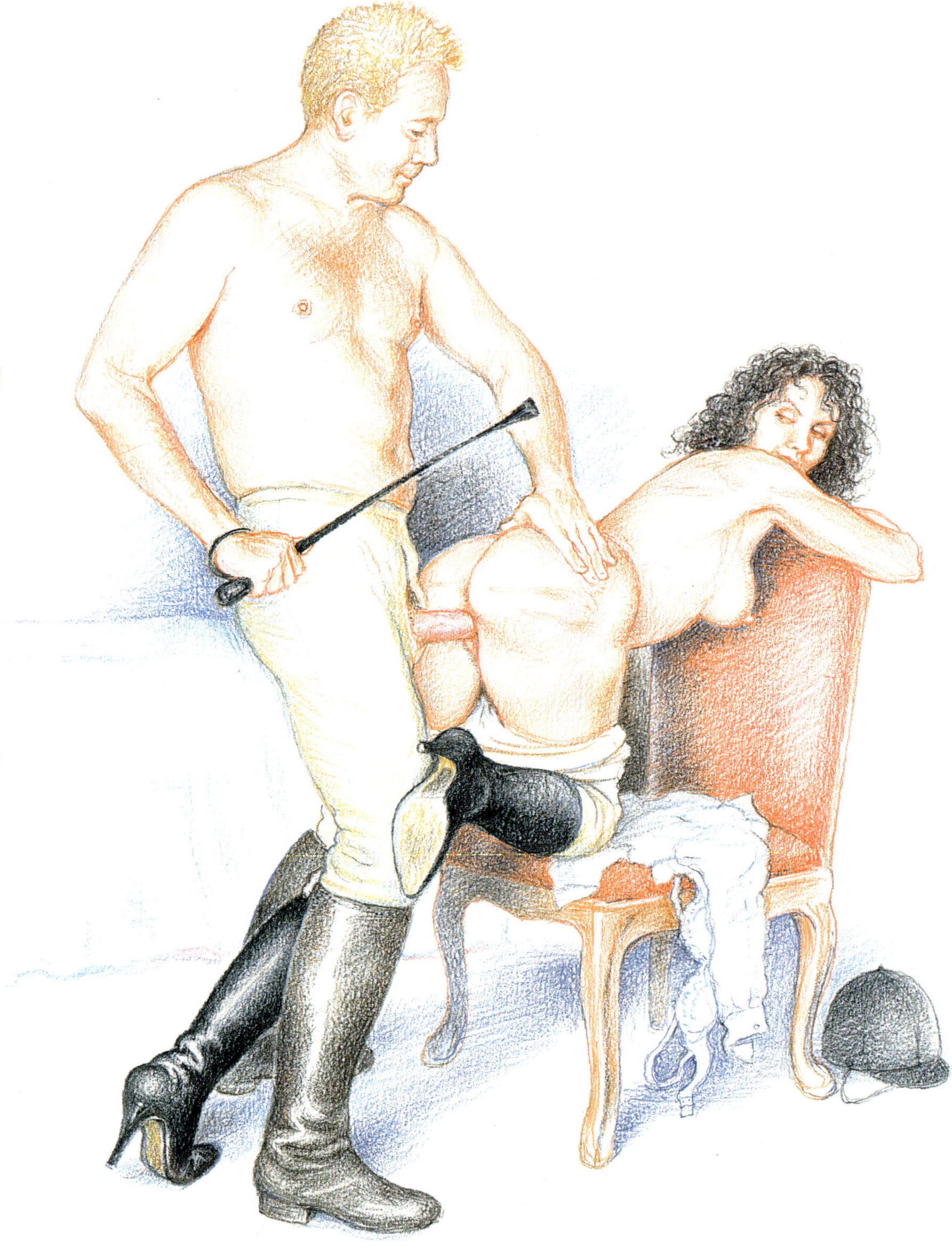

The Riding Crop

A man's leather slipper is ideal. It makes a nice 'thwack' and delivers a good sting but will do no damage because it is not long enough. A leather belt can be more difficult to control, and hurt more because of its length. I would not recommend it. Then we have hairbrushes (use the back surface, not the prickly side), wooden spoons and plastic rulers. Some hairbrushes are good if there is enough handle to get hold of, but wooden spoons must be approached with caution as they can pack a punch and be quite alarmingly painful! Always be cautious with anything metal, like kitchen spatulas.

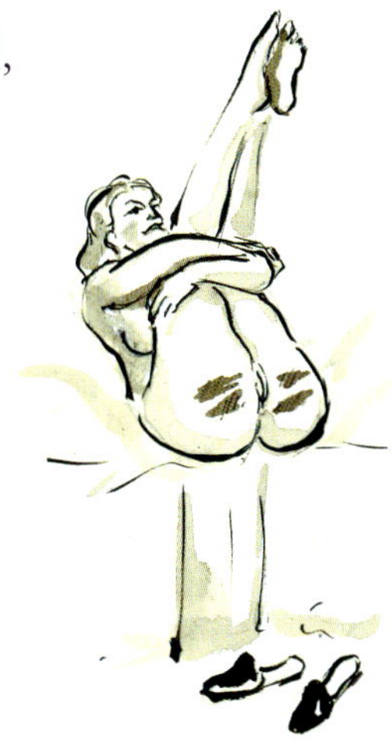

Slipper Spank

The hairbrush is a splendid implement for using when you have your naughty brat over your knee and have easy access to the bedroom dressing table, and likewise the plastic ruler if you happen to be punishing your male or female miscreant in the office, but some of you might enjoy to visit a specialist shop or fetish fair to select a professionally made implement that will feel more erotic to use (see section on visiting a sex shop together, p. 98). It is all a matter of your personal preference – some prefer to reach for whatever comes to hand in the domestic environment, while others prefer the beautifully made implement which is tucked away lovingly in a special drawer and *only* used for the specific purpose of warming someone's bottom.

For those who feel attracted to the atmosphere of school chastisements, the appropriate implements will be the tawse, the strap, the paddle and the cane – all rather formidable in their own way. I'd like to leave aside the cane for the moment, for although this is the implement above all others which conjures up for most of us the traditional visit to the headmaster's study (whether we have ever experienced real CP at school or not), it is not an instrument to be trifled with. Only the most dedicated devotees will wish to experiment with it for it needs practice and care.

Let us return to Lucy Bailey, the expert on implements:

Straps and paddles come in a multitude of different shapes and intensities. Paddles generally have a distinct handle whereas straps do not. Tawses are basically straps that have one or two splits to create fingers cut into the end. These implements are most suited for use on bottoms, tops of legs and hands. Straps and tawses are generally made from leather while paddles can come in a variety of different finishes such as leather, rubber, plastic and wood. I prefer these classic implements when made from quality leather. There is something quite delicious about the feel of leather against the skin.

Paddles tend to cover a bigger area of the bottom than a strap and since they are usually stiff you don't have to worry about controlling the tip as much. When using straps or tawses you should measure the stroke before delivering it. To measure the stroke use a technique where the first strike you make merely touches the bottom gently. You can then check where the stroke has landed and thus ensure you know exactly where a hard strike will land. Ensure that the tip of the implement lands about three-quarters of the way into the furthest buttock.

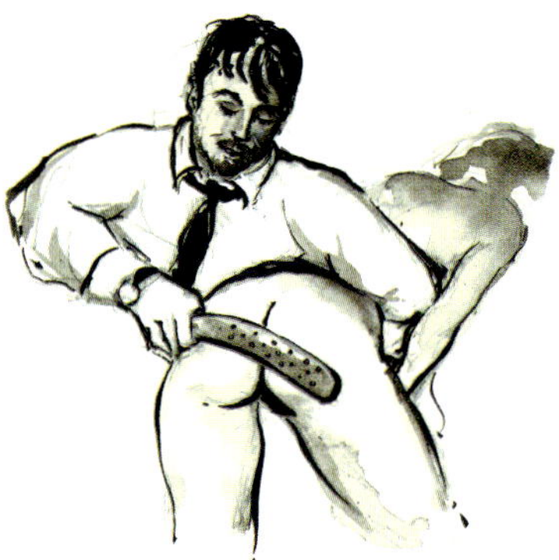

The longer the strap the harder it is to control the tip, so the more practice you need before using it. Try to get the flat of the strap or tawse and not the edge to land on the bottom or target area. It should land with a good crack if it lands correctly and a dull sound if wrong. I have found the main problem when receiving strokes from these

implements is that the furthest buttock can continually receive all the punishment. As the Dominant it is important to be aware of this problem as it concentrates the pain onto one area making the beating uncomfortable in the wrong way! To solve this problem I would suggest either aim and strike at each cheek separately or alternate with a backhand stroke so that each cheek receives the same amount of punishment.

Well, I bet you didn't realise that there was so much to it… Lucy is quite right. I can speak from my own experience here: there are certain types of pain, mainly brought about by lack of skill, which can cause the recipient real anguish and make them tense with fear of what is to come next. This is not what any submissive really wants.

Now we come to riding crops and whips.

Riding crops are fibreglass rods covered in leather or nylon mesh-weave. They end in some kind of leather tip. The tip of a riding crop, the keeper, is usually either two flaps or a single loop of leather. This was designed to make a loud noise as the two pieces of leather slap together and thus spur on the horse. They come in a huge variety of designs. The standard length is 28 inches although you can find longer and shorter ones. Riding crops are easy to buy from riding shops and saddleries.

When buying a crop it must have *a large tip, the keeper at the end; this should be of at least one inch square or larger and made with a reasonably heavy piece of leather. Some crops have hand shapes at the end and others rubber tips, though rubber is a little too biting for my taste.*

I feel I can best explain from experience how pleasurable it can be to receive a crop stroke properly and how painful and off-putting it is to receive a bad one. A bad stroke usually comes when someone attempts to use the riding crop like a cane. IT ISN'T A CANE! Unlike a cane it has a knot at the end that holds the tip/fall in place. If the shaft of the whip or the knot hits you it is most unpleasant and there is no nice crack – just a dull thud and a deep painful indentation where the knot has probably cut into your skin. A good stroke is where only the tip hits you. Being a doubled piece of leather it should make a lovely crack which actually sounds a little worse than it is. As both a giver and receiver I actually find this sound quite erotic and, as I have said, a good indication to the effectiveness of the shot.

WHIPS

I agree with Lucy that the unique sound of your favourite whip can be an immense turn-on. This brings us to the category of multi-stranded whips, implements of great versatility and to my mind, the most erotic.

Whips come in various sizes depending on the length of the thongs, which come in just about every finish: leather, rubber, suede, pigskin, rope. The material of the thongs will usually determine how soft or hard the whip is. Multiple whips have either flat or rounded tails. Thongs can range in length from 6 to 26 inches. Much longer than this and they become very difficult to handle. My personal interpretation is that those with round, stingy thongs are known as 'cats', while whips with flat thongs are called 'floggers'.

A well known implement is the French 'martinet', although strangely there is no such thing in the English dictionary. A martinet is a 'strict disciplinarian' rather than an actual implement. What is often called a martinet is really a type of 'cat' with a cylindrical wooden handle and around eight to twelve long, thin, round tails.

Whips have the capacity and advantage of being able to cover a large area. They can be used on most of the body but are particularly effective for flogging the back and bottom. When beating the back care should be taken not to strike the spine or the kidney area directly.

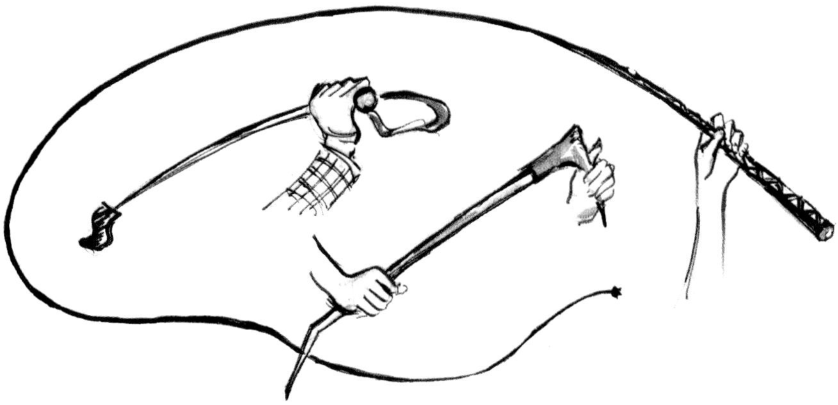

Whips Selection

We will talk more of this kind of whip in the next section for on the whole these are not the sort of implements most associated with traditional CP. Whenever you are buying any sort of implement, always make sure they are strong and well-made and test that they feel right in your hand.

THE CANE

The most difficult implement of all to use is probably the cane. For me, this implement is so closely associated with cruelties inflicted on youngsters in our traditional English education system up until the 1950s, and in some cases even later, that I personally find it hard to link it with eroticism, but I can assure you that given the right situation and with an expert in charge it can be used to good effect as a climax to any CP session.

No two canes are ever identical, as they are natural products; grown, not manufactured. There is an endless variety of rattans of varying thicknesses, lengths, curvature, flexibility and colour. Some are crook-handled and some are straight. Here is more helpful advice from Lucy:

I would suggest that a beginner use a short, lightweight cane. The longer the cane the more swing, the greater the arc, equalling a more painful stroke. Remember the longer the cane the more difficult it is to control. The weight of the cane changes the sensation and intensity of the stroke. The thinner the cane the more 'stingy' and biting it feels. While thicker canes are heavier, more 'thumpy' and tend to bruise the skin. With more weight they penetrate more deeply.

Caning is probably one of the most revered of the disciplinary arts taking some time to perfect. A perfect cane stroke needs a minimum amount of effort, you don't have to throw your whole body into it. In fact the greatest accuracy is achieved with the minimum variation of movement. This is probably one of the reasons why the cane is such a favoured disciplinary tool. The stature and strength of the disciplinarian is immaterial as it is one's technique that is all-important (the cane is certainly a great equaliser for women). Before beginning a punishment with the cane it is really advisable to have a thorough warm-up to help prevent serious bruises and cuts. Despite appearances canes are very severe implements, so NEVER USE FULL FORCE BLOWS as they may cause damage to underlying tissue and nerves.

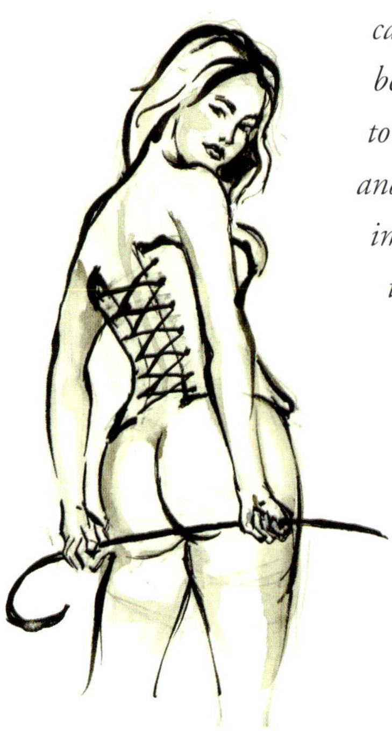

Lucy goes on to advise us that the safest and most accurate technique for using the cane is the 'wrist only' movement:

Hold the cane in your hand, tuck your elbow into your body and using only your lower arm, use a fast wrist motion to flick the cane at the target. If you cane without moving your wrist you cannot get any speed into the motion of the stroke or that lovely 'swish' noise, as you are not really using the flexibility of the cane.

Always aim at the fleshy part of the buttocks; I cannot stress this enough, for accidentally striking someone too high up near the base of their spine can be agony for them, not to mention dangerous. You are walking a tightrope here between intense pleasure at one end of the spectrum and totally un-erotic pain at the other which can become an instant turn-off. Please don't take any risks.

Bringing us back to a lighter note, dressing up can heighten one's enjoyment of these scenes, but more of that later. There is also a variety of positions we can use for chastising, making full use of the everyday furniture you have in your home. Instead of describing each one, you can get some ideas by perusing magazines and possibly think of a few for yourselves.

We haven't yet mentioned that important question of rituals to heighten the sense of anticipation. The one to be punished will quickly be made aware that the scenario has begun when they hear the change of voice in their partner. A good way to heighten the feeling of nervous expectation further is to tell them to go and fetch the implement to be used on them from its special cupboard, bring it and present it properly to the Master or Mistress. Lucy has this to add:

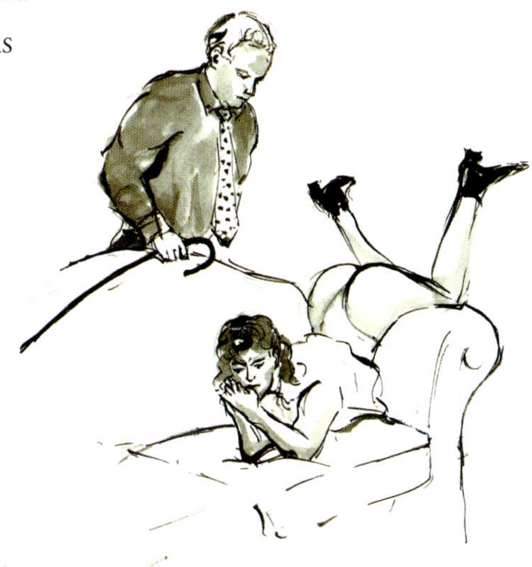

Letting the offender know of their punishment in advance is often very much a part of the discipline itself. It draws the punishment out longer. You can

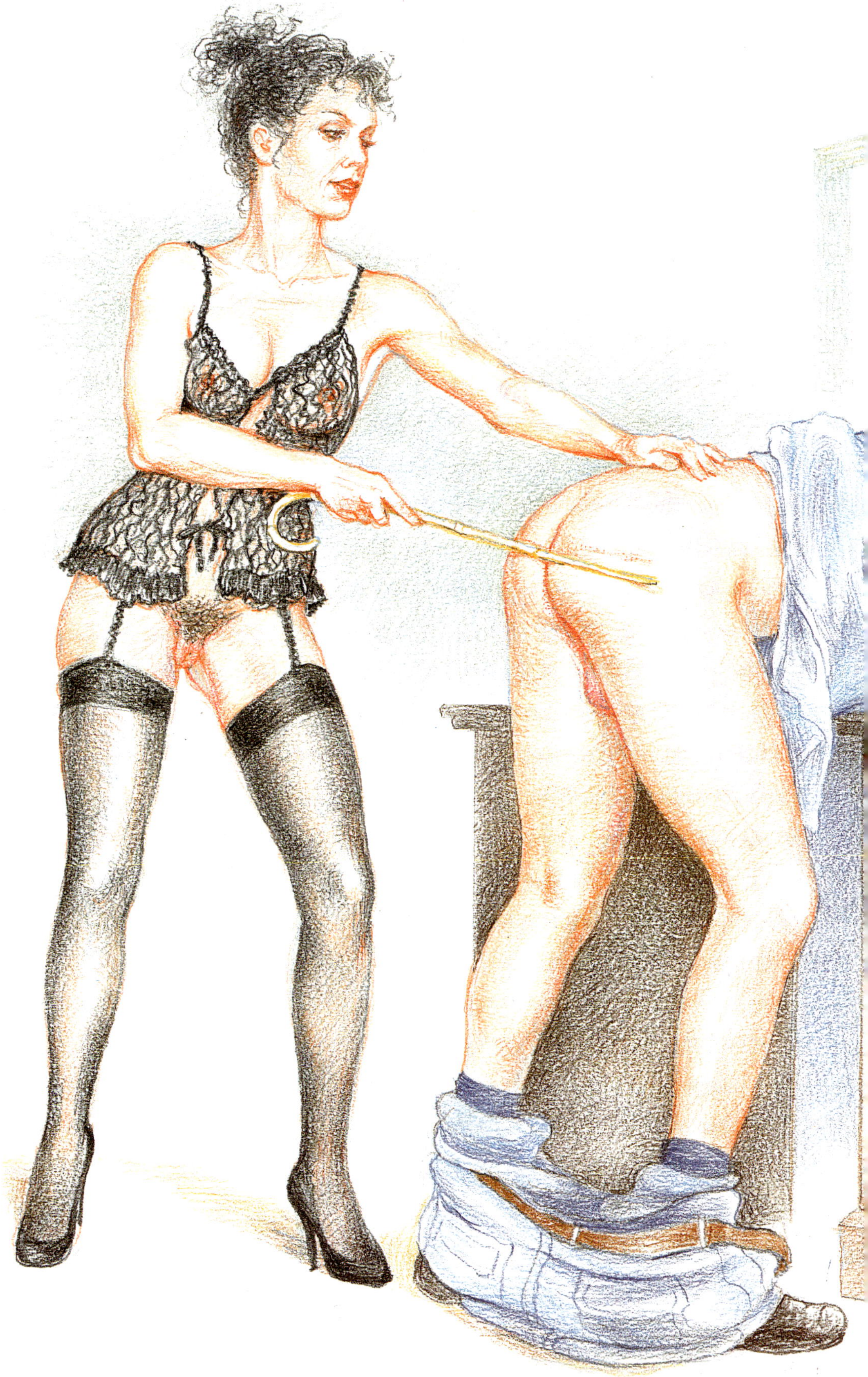

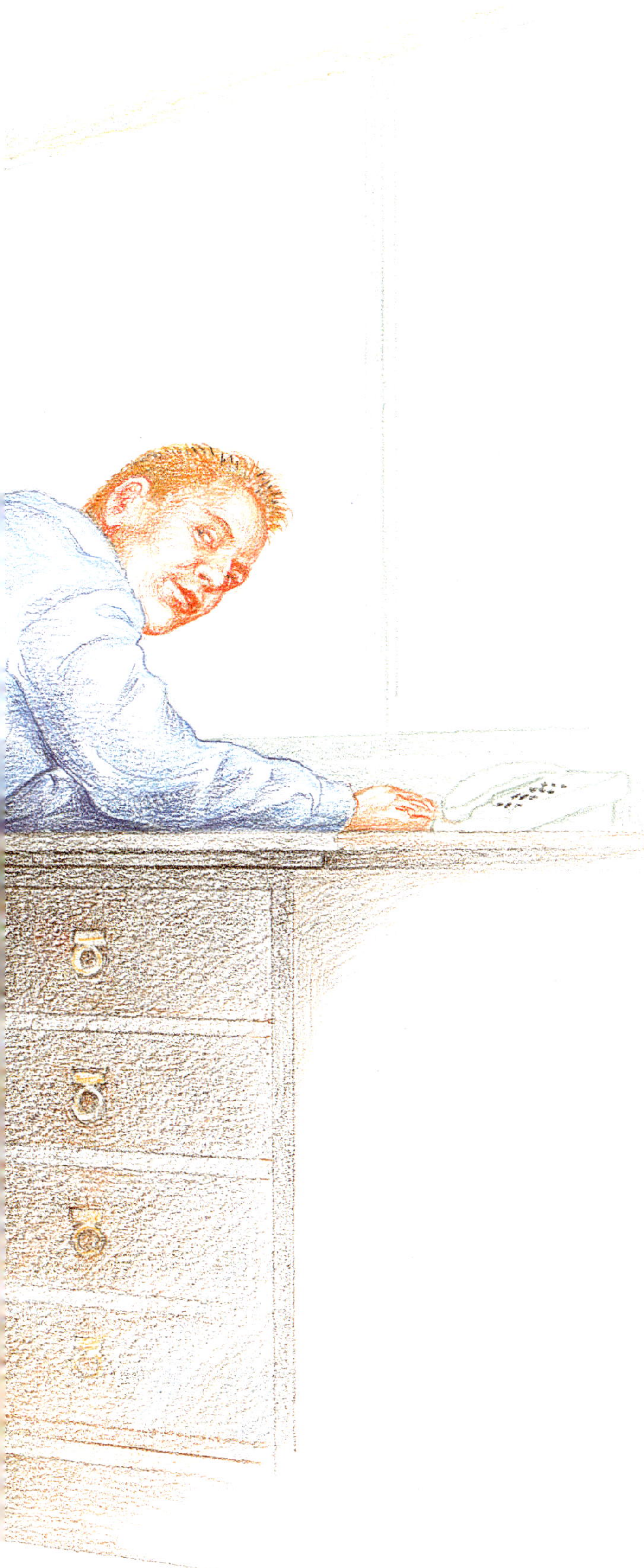

Always aim at the fleshy
part of the buttocks

announce the day and time the discipline will be dished out, what they should wear, what implement and how many.

Lucy then goes on to mention the keeping of a punishment book and how exciting that can be. It can be particularly handy if there is a reason why you can't attend to the spanking straight away (maybe you have visitors, or the children are there). The book can be discreetly written in and the miscreant will know what they have coming.

There could be a tariff of what punishments will be given out for what misdemeanours. The book can then be called upon during a scene so that the submissive is actually punished for real mistakes.

During a real punishment I can go through different emotions, feeling that it is unfair, or feeling guilty about my actions and wanting to be really punished hard for them. For smaller misdemeanours I personally have found an instant slap or immediate spanking probably one of the most sexually fulfilling experiences I have. When these happen they are real. They do not turn into sex and are genuine chastisements where I am left feeling contrite and penitent.

I think real punishments within any relationship are amazingly cathartic and work especially well within close relationships... When I am rude or snappy and my partner does not respond I feel guilty and he feels annoyed with me. However, if I am smacked or punished I think we both feel much better. I must point out that this probably wouldn't work during a blazing row. I do not think it is ever really a good idea to enter into any sub/dom games when either partner is really angry or out of control. They can of course be written into the book and dealt with at a later stage when things are a little calmer.

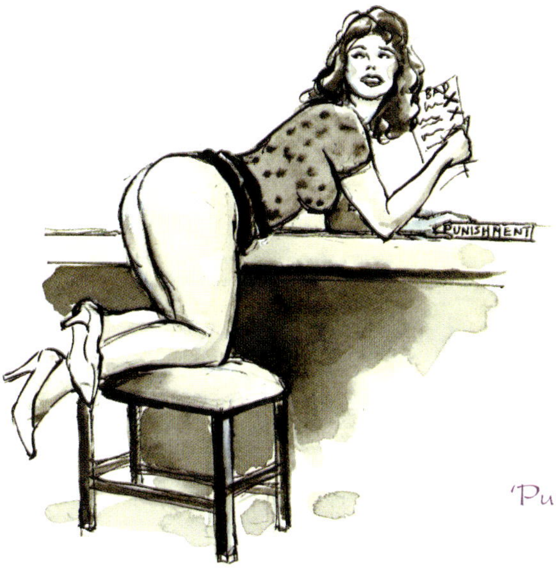

Some couples find the 'Punishment Book' a good way to build erotic tension

The times when I have been beaten for real (nothing to do with sex), I have become incredibly sexually excited almost to the point of orgasm. I suppose the instantaneous action makes the whole punishment real. (Plus, of course, the sensation of a glowing bottom and the exhilaration from all the squirming around). Nonetheless, I believe it is something much more than that and difficult to explain. I think that beating someone can be an incredibly loving act. The dominant wants what is best for his or her partner… CP can become an act of love and care, which creates a very close bond between the disciplinarian and the recipient.

All this may seem an odd business to those uninitiated ones and believe me, I can sympathise with your feelings. I once had an unforgettable conversation with a man over a dinner table who was telling me how he attached great value to the use of the whip in his relations with his wife. Being an inexperienced young woman at the time I was somewhat taken

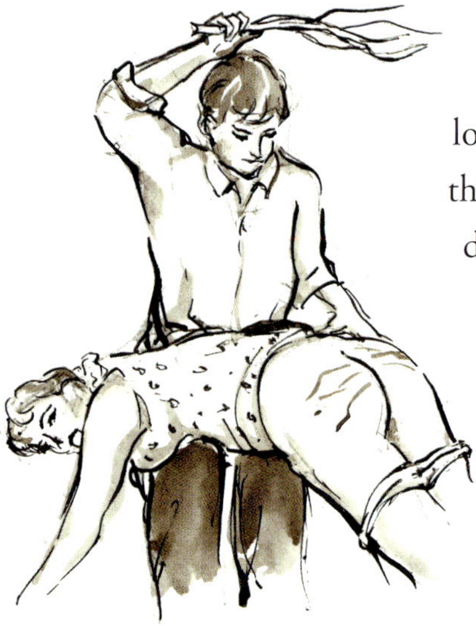

Using the Birch

aback that this subject could be discussed so openly with the gentleman's wife sitting there looking demure and inscrutable. But I had to admit that I began to be immensely intrigued as he described the rituals they had evolved and the erotic adventures they had both enjoyed together. He cast his eyes towards the wall where an array of leather paddles, martinets and whips were hanging. 'They are the tools of transformation,' he informed me, and that description has always stayed in my mind.

Only much later did I begin to get an inkling of what he meant.

There has to be a purpose to all these rituals, separating them from anything which smacks of abuse and real cruelty. This is a safe and controlled way to explore the greater depths of a relationship and must always be enjoyed by both parties and entered into with sincerity and trust.

Let's close this section by hearing from a male spanking enthusiast now and let him have the last word on the subject:

To many it's the thrill of apparently being helpless whilst under the complete control of their partner, yet knowing that in actual fact it's the person being spanked that runs the game. To some it's the pleasure of watching their partner's bottom bouncing wildly under their descending hand. It can also be the afterglow one feels after the spanking is over. This is different for everybody and simply has to be experienced.

The joy of both of you looking into a mirror afterwards and observing the transformation from a once pale naked bottom to a piece of glowing, blushing, poetry in vision is an experience not to be missed.

The thing that to me sets spanking aside from all other forms of CP is the infinite variety of role-plays which are possible. No props need to be used. No expensive equipment. One frequently used is the Teacher/Naughty Pupil scenario. Infinite varieties in this one, which can involve dressing up. Wouldn't you like to see your female partner in her old, or newly acquired school uniform? With her tie badly fastened, and her socks loose round her ankles? With regulation blue, green or brown knickers just waiting to be pulled down, and her naughty young bottom soundly spanked? Maybe the acquisition of a mortarboard and gown? This can easily be done in reverse of course, with the tutor or headmistress pulling the protesting schoolboy over her lap and giving him the treatment he so richly deserves. So many variations. Doctor and nurse, overspending partner, rude shop assistant. You could try writing the first ever spanking play (if either or both of you are dramatically inclined), or use card or other games where the loser gets spanked.

One word of caution: I would strongly advise against any real area of contention coming into your role-play; keep it in the imagination. The most important thing to remember here is that all CP enthusiasts will call themselves players, and playing is exactly what it is, or should be.

Implements? Yes, they can be used, and can add to the fun (hairbrushes, wooden spatulas and the like). Remember, though, these are not as controllable as hands, and can hurt more, so use with caution at first.

Does it lead to lovemaking? Frequently. But it doesn't have to. It can be enjoyed for its own sake.

Safe words: There must always be a safe word, known to both parties. This should ideally be something totally disassociated from the game in hand. It would not be possible to miss something like RED SOCKS! or TEDDY

BEARS! or something like that. On hearing this, the spanker must stop, certainly for the moment.

This is most important to remember, the 'spankee', or 'bottom', must be ultimately in charge. Also, I believe that the spanker should have been spanked at some time. This is the only way you can know how much pain you are inflicting on your partner. Of course you may have a bum like leather and your partner have a very low pain threshold, but at least it will be some guide.

A TOUCH OF PAIN AS STIMULATION

Not everyone responds to the idea of punishment and contrition but they may still wish to stretch the boundaries of sensations a little wider. To me, understanding the way our nerves and senses work and giving them a heightened erotic stimulus from time to time is like adding a wider spectrum of colour and tone to a painting, deepening its shadows and touching the highlights with a dab of brilliant white.

Usually, the immediate response to feeling pain of any sort is to feel personally affronted as if whatever caused this assault on our nerve endings did it with the express intention of hurting us. Usually we can't help feeling this – even if the offender is an inanimate object that we have clumsily banged into. If we can only separate ourselves off from this automatic reaction and accept these sensual gradations, from pastel shades to dazzlingly brilliant colours, then there will be a change in the way we experience them. As I said earlier, where there is trust and a desire to embrace new things, the more painful aspects can heighten our intensity of involvement and flow through us in a different way.

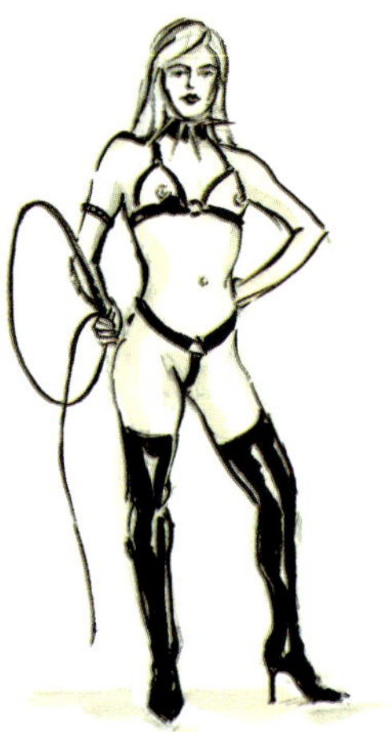

To start with, whipping does not have to be done in a harsh, punitive way. There are various techniques for handling a whip purely to arouse your partner (see illustration), and you can find some beautiful, soft implements on the market, made from material like pig-skin or suede, that cannot damage the skin, even when used with force. One of my favourites has tails of flat thongs measuring about 6 inches long attached by studs to a handle of roughly the same length. It can be used over the whole body and because it is short it can be easily controlled and used on places where you wouldn't generally consider using a whip at all, like the nipples.

Whipping women's breasts with anything hard is definitely not recommended, but if you would like to try a safer and much more erotic method which will get even the most reticent pair of nipples standing up to attention, strip naked and stand with your legs a little apart for balance, and your hands behind your head. This will ensure that your breasts are forced up and outwards. Then get your partner to bring down the soft whip carefully so that only the tips of the thongs catch your nipple, giving it an invigorating sting. If this is pleasurable, then the whipping can be continued down your body to your stomach and work round the thighs to your bottom and back (even with this soft whip I would still advise you not to touch the base of the spine; it's best to acquire safe habits).

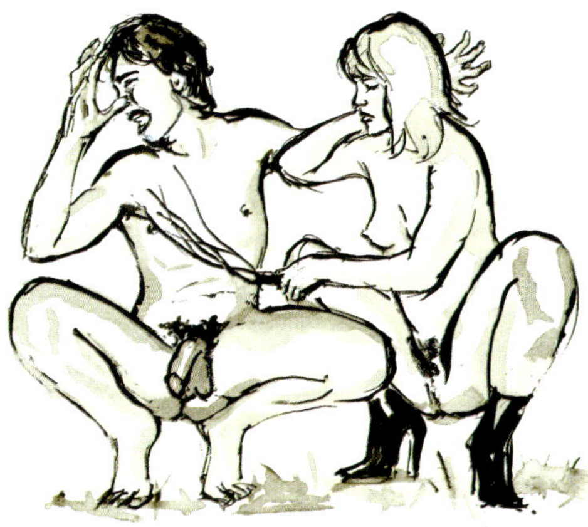

Nipple Whipping

To go to town on a really erotic whipping experience you must cast your mind back to those first experiments we talked about earlier where you collected all the paraphernalia for sensual delights from feathers to ice cubes. Have all these items ready and put them together with your newly acquired selection of whips. Dim the lights (or light some scented candles), put on your favourite sensual music, and both of you get naked. Then one of you is blindfolded and lies face down on the bed. Place a cushion or pillow under their bottom to present it nicely for the treatment, but make sure that they are completely comfortable before you begin.

Start by massaging your partner all over their body, warming the muscles and relaxing the tension, all the while talking quietly to them. As you get more deeply into the massage, drag your nails lightly down their back (taking care to avoid any moles they might have) and across their buttocks, interspersed with kisses, nibbles and licks of the tongue here and there. When you feel they are ready, reach for a whip with long, soft tails and start to drag it sensually over them, tickling and caressing them, running the tails between their legs. Then change to one with shorter tails and start to flick the whip, starting lightly and slowly at first then building up the stinging sensations, covering them all over and increasing the pace. These soft whips can also be made to whirr in a circular motion which can be exciting provided you stay well clear of the face and neck. If you also have a crop with a large soft tip, you can start to tap them sharply with that, using just the end, gradually increasing the severity of the taps until their flesh tingles.

Now whisper in their ear and get your lover to turn over, continuing the flicking on their front. Stop to lick, tweak or bite a nipple, increasing the severity until they are standing up, then flick the stiffened nipples with the soft whip, or the tip of the crop. Make sure their whole body is stimulated: arms, legs and sides as well as the insides of their thighs. Just keep going and don't rush. As their skin warms and becomes flushed with a lovely pink your partner will be able to take more stings and slaps from the implements. If this is really working for them their arousal will become apparent. (I don't need to tell you that if it isn't, that will be apparent too.) When someone needs more whipping in a certain area they tend to push that part of their body towards the whip, welcoming it.

It is not generally thought of, but light whipping can be used to get the blood flowing to the genitals too. For use on your woman, you need to find an implement thoroughly suited to the job. It needs to be a very small, light paddle, with a hard handle and tongue consisting of a single thickness of soft leather no more than six inches long. When she is lying back comfortably (you can leave the pillow under her bottom to make sure her pussy is properly presented to you) start to strike downwards (gently at first) with the implement, around the inside of the tops of her thighs, moving in carefully to land it on the area on and around her clitoris. Bear in mind that not all women can get enjoyment from this form of stimulation, but try it for a few minutes, varying the severity of the strokes and see how she takes to it. When attempting something new it is always wise to remember the way you get the temperature of a shower to suit you: start off cool and then gradually run the hot water in until it is just right. Stop at once if it isn't working. I know this technique does cause pleasurable writhings in some, indeed I have even watched with amazement as a girlfriend of mine was 'pussy-whipped' to powerful orgasm, but it doesn't necessarily please all of us in the same way.

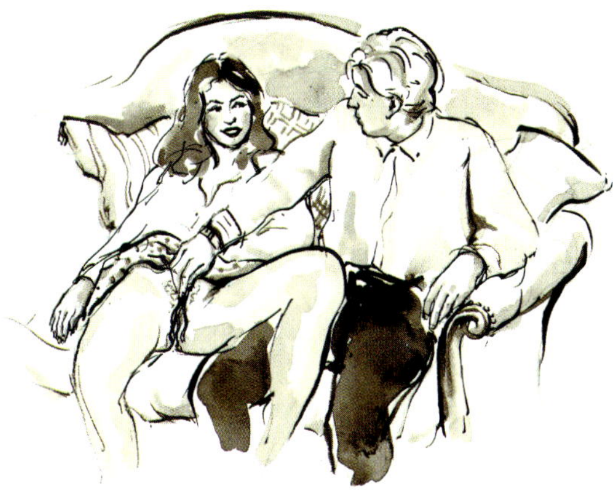

'Pussy Whipping'

If you want to try the whip on a willing

cock then use the short, soft-tailed whip. If he is lying down, cup one hand over his balls first, for there is nothing worse than being caught a stinging blow in that delicate region – you could put him off for life; then circle your thumb and forefinger around the base of his shaft as it lies across his belly and use the gentle flicking motions on the underside of his penis. Or, to make it easier for you, ask him to protect himself with his own hands and make his penis stand up so that you can whip him all round.

Erotic whippings can be a wonderfully arousing part of foreplay and because there is no dominant/submissive scenario, you can swap around and try out different sensations on each other. If you know that your nipples are especially sensitive and play a big part in arousing you, then you will probably respond to some intense treatment with nipple clamps. There are several kinds of these, of varying severity, available from most good sex shops. Some have little teeth, and some are like clothes pegs, but all work on a similar principle to the clip-on earring. Again, as with whipping, you need to be warmed up nicely first. After a bit of your favourite foreplay, suck the nipple to make it stand up then pinch it very near its base so that it sticks out as far as possible and carefully apply the clamps to bite on as much of the nipple as possible, but take it slowly; some clamps can be agonising. When they are in place they will draw attention to your throbbing nipples constantly and as you get more aroused the pain will become more bearable.

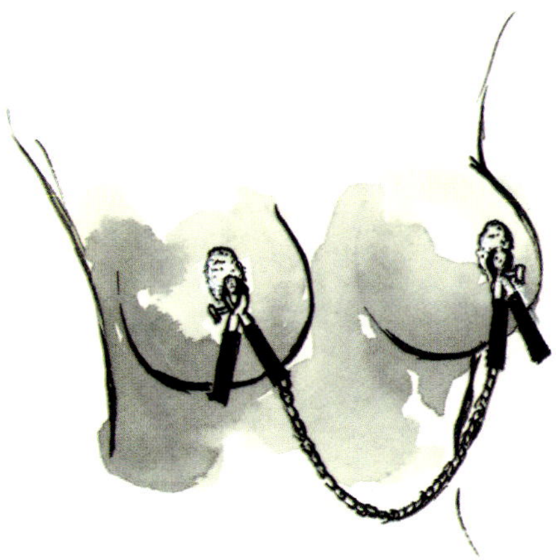

Nipple Clamps

Some clamps are attached to a chain which means that you can take hold of it and pull tantalisingly to increase the 'suffering' of the tortured one. Why not have him on his back, make him hard and then sit on top of his cock, gently easing him in. While you fuck him you can give a little tug on the chain when you want to 'gee him up' (not too much, or the clamps will come off) as if it were a rein. Having his hands bound and kept out of the way for this will increase his feeling of helplessness.

A woman's nipples are usually larger than a man's so there is a bigger area for attaching the clamps and they are less likely to fall off. Some devotees like to use weighted clamps so that there is a constant dragging sensation and if you kneel on all fours, gravity will cause your breasts to stretch out in an amazing fashion. To be taken from behind with the weights dangling and swaying like pendulums from your breasts is a truly unique experience!

Be aware that the greatest pain from strong nipple clamps comes when they are removed and will be worse the longer they remain on. For a very memorable, albeit brief agony, allow the clamps to be pulled off, but if this is likely to be over the top for you, very, very slowly unclip the clamps yourself. When they are off, the pain surges briefly and then subsides, leaving you with two wonderfully enlarged throbbing nipples.

Less scary clips can be attached to the inner labia of the vagina allowing your partner to pull the lips apart using the chains. Some devotees enjoy the weighted clamps and love to feel their lips being stretched downwards when they stand with their feet apart. If this is sexily exciting for you, it is very likely you will enjoy being shaved and pierced too, but more on that later.

Talking of piercing, for those who cannot get enough of the nipple attention, a large needle can be used delicately to prick the nipple itself, giving exquisite sensations, but never try to pierce too deeply (if you want

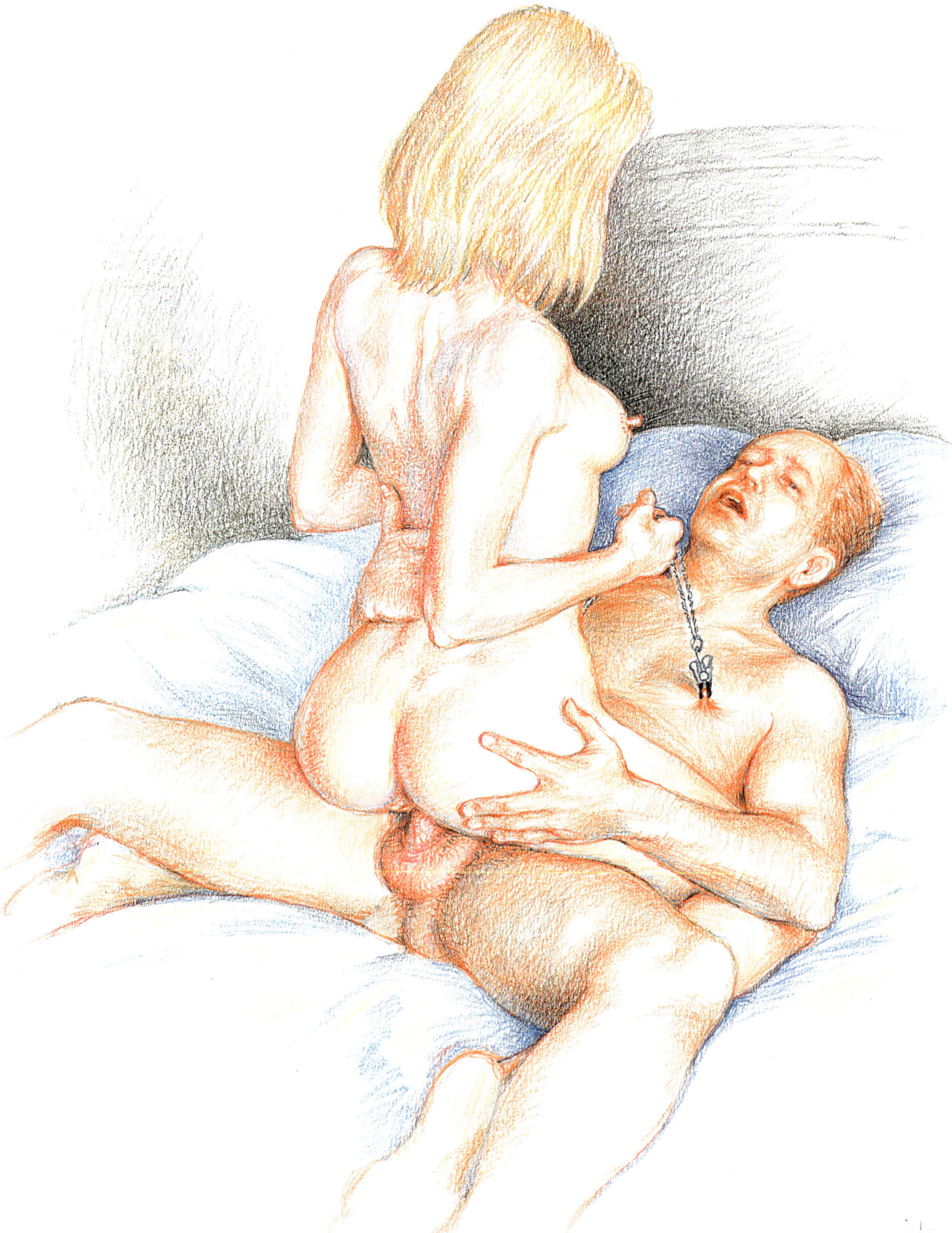

Giving a Tug to
Gee Him Up

to be really pierced, get it done properly by a professional). Needles should always be sterilised by dipping in alcohol or holding in a flame.

Another way of producing a short, sharp twinge of pain with no harmful after-effects is to drip hot wax direct from a candle onto the skin (avoid genitals for this) but make sure the candle is no nearer than a foot away. The wax needs that split second, as it drops through the air, to cool just a little bit.

The purpose in this section is not to mention everything that can be done, for some enthusiasts of the SM scene will think up many surprising and sometimes dangerous ways of giving painful shocks to each other and I have no intention of going into those realms. Once you have a few basic things that work for both of you, the challenge is to think of imaginative and different ways of using them. The aim should not be to challenge yourself further and further; a greater pain or protracted punishment does not necessarily lead to a greater degree of excitement and a more powerful orgasm. That sort of attitude leads to a dead end. The true fulfilment comes from the joy of expressing yourself.

LIGHT BONDAGE: DUNGEONS AND EQUIPMENT

Bondage is the act of restricting a person's movement, and in my experience there are few who don't find this physically arousing, whether they admit it or not.

Historically, bondage was used on stolen brides, to prevent their escape. This restraint evolved into symbolic bindings, such as ties around the waist or the ankles and wrists.

There is even a school of thought that the wedding ring is a remaining symbol of that bondage, but we can't be sure about this. Certainly, the custom of carrying a bride over the threshold originates from the days

The secret life of a female submissive

My interest in SM developed from very early childhood fantasies. They are not much to do with actual punishments received from adults but more peer role play activity and fantasy ideas. I was very well treated at home, and corporal punishment featured very little in my home and school life. I did watch television programs, for instance 'Billy Bunter', which may have shaped my expectations, but the idea of restraints, sexual punishments and the thrill of exposure began before age three.

My earliest recollection is of a self-inflicted bondage experiment, where I discovered that pushing both my feet through my teething ring held my ankles tightly together and was very difficult to get off – I found this erotically exciting, especially when sitting on my pot in the dark. My first playmate, a little boy a few months younger than myself, was the earliest great love of my life. We were friends from early babyhood and were together almost every weekday until I started school at the age of four and a half. We were lovers, so far as we understood it then, often kissing and cuddling, and I introduced him to a 'game' which involved exposing our bare bottoms in anticipation that we were being naughty and would be spanked. We also took turns to tie each other up – in cowboy and Indian games – when we were a little older, about six or seven.

I lost contact with this particular friend when we went on to different schools and my SM interests were then indulged only in private, alone

when a bride couldn't walk across the threshold because she was tied up.

From childhood, we use bondage for fun and in games: cowboys and Indians, spies and secret agents, and so on. I'm not the only one to have felt a definite – if at the time uninterpretable – frisson at being 'caught' by the enemy and tied to a chair. But now we are all grown up, bondage can be even more fun.

What an individual gets out of bondage is a personal thing; you will know, in your heart of hearts, whether you are a bondage 'top' (i.e. if you like being in charge, you like to structure the play) or if you are a 'bottom' (i.e. you like to be tied, to be the 'object' of the play). Very many people, in the realm of light bondage, are what is known as 'switches' (i.e. they like a little of both).

For those who are 'bottoms' there is in store the wonderful release of inhibition that comes with being tied up. Whatever happens to you while you are bound is not your responsibility. You are (in theory) helpless to stop it and so you can simply give in and enjoy it. Luxuriate in the absolute lack of control and let go.

Men – because they, in general, are stronger than their partner – often enjoy the way their restriction equalises the physical relationship, or even gives the woman the upper hand. This can be very sexy but, like absolutely everything else, only if both partners are comfortable with the scenario and the power dynamic within it.

There is a great deal of trust involved in bondage – as in all BD/SM games. The 'bottom' reaps the benefits of that trust in being able to surrender without fear and the 'top' reaps the benefits in being given a licence to luxuriate in total control over another human being. For the duration of the game, a 'top' has a feeling of incredible personal power – you can touch but not be touched, see and not be seen, hear but not be heard. You can do everything you want and yet control exactly how much your partner can do. It can be sexually exhilarating.

Some people enjoy the use of blindfolds with bondage – somehow the

and secretly – I would tie myself up with belts, especially tightly between the legs and around my thighs and waist. I would beat myself with a strap. I also liked to 'trap' myself by hanging over the banisters naked, taking risks of being seen naked in the garden, etc. The joint practices of CP and bondage appealed to me especially, but unaware that other people did such things, I believed I was perhaps the only one. I would also subject myself to ice-cold water and then very hot water alternately on my genitals. (Actually no one else has ever done this to me, nor a number of other things that I still do privately occasionally). I masturbated as far back as I can remember, but again did not know that others did this. It was not until I was 13 that I learned what masturbation was and that others did it.

So far as a deeper understanding of SM developing, at 19 I started to read 'Forum' magazine and discovered that there were others who liked similar activities, and later, at 26, I began to experiment with SM-type scenarios with my then husband, who unfortunately did not find it interesting. At 33 I became acquainted with the SM club scene and met my current master when I was 36. I am now 50.

I would not describe pleasure in the stimulation of pain as straightforward because it seems to be highly variable – what is pleasurable one day may not be so the next; levels ebb and flow. For me, pain needs to be combined with restraint in some form – physical or mental. Role play can be fun because it sets up a fantasy

built and this in itself is sufficient 'restraint' for me as it is almost impossible to escape from his hold. We always keep a few implements to hand for spontaneous sessions – small riding crops, cat whips (which are quite soft and sensual), paddles – beside the bed, and others around the living room. When nothing is handy, improvisation occurs e.g. wooden spoons in the kitchen, a ruler from the desk. These are playful scenes which can spark up in a moment and be over fairly quickly. There is another side to both of us which emerges at other times and makes for a more concentrated scene. This is very much a mood thing – the one in the mood becomes quiet, but is also restless and broody, and a bit snappy. There is a 'floppiness' and a tendency to adopt submissive postures when touched (a bit like the way a cat responds when stroked). This is the sign for a more intense scene which usually happens in bed, with some teasing and CP, and will end with intercourse. As a general rule we prefer not to wear a lot of clothing indoors, and my partner often removes his trousers when sitting by the fire in the evenings. I may kneel in front of him and then embrace his legs and body in an affectionate, submissive gesture. This often will initiate further action, and can go in a number of directions as the mood suggests. We also enjoy sex without any SM foreplay, but it is certainly true of both of us that we are using SM fantasies in our imaginations to reach orgasm. Some therapists recommend that couples should discuss these fantasies together but we have not found this helpful – in fact it has even had the

of mine who makes whips for a living makes wonderful leather cuffs that are tightened and attached by means of long leather ties.

You can also get leather ankle cuffs that are joined by a metal bar. When worn, they have the effect of spreading your legs without them having to be bound to anything else (useful on the 'meathook' – see below). Most decent sex shops have a reasonable selection… just don't be shy about examining them. After all – you could be wearing them a lot!

The only thing I really don't like are handcuffs. The fur-lined ones are a bit silly and non-fur-lined ones downright uncomfortable. Unless it is in a role-play situation involving nasty policemen or policewomen, there are so many better ways to bind someone.

And now – you need to find a position that works for you

I have a friend who loves to be tied up with arms above her head so that she is standing right up on tiptoe. Her partner calls it the 'meathook'. Although this is a distinctly unappealing term, it is a very sexy position. Sexy for the 'top' because they have your whole body stretched out for them to do anything they want to it`. They can stroke and pinch, lick and nibble – everywhere is accessible to them. And it's sexy for the 'bottom' too, because you *know* you look great stretched out like that; what's more, there's a real feeling of exposure and helplessness as you hang there.

Starting like this you can progress down the BD/SM route and start whipping or spanking… or you can simply have wonderful sex standing up.

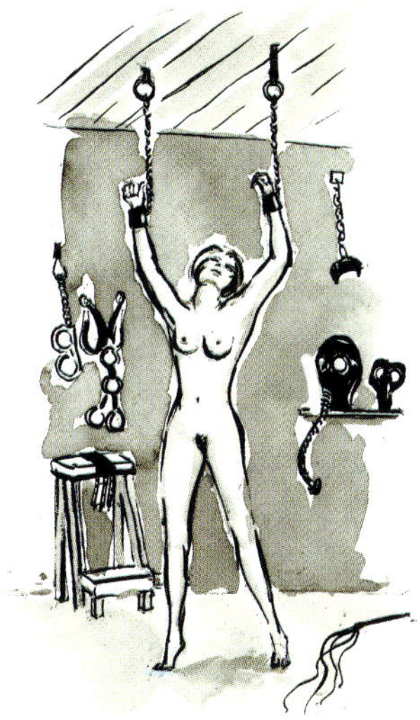

disappointing effect of 'desensualising' the fantasy, or causing disappointment for the partner in feeling that they are inadequate!

What sort of things turn me on particularly? Buttock spanking, riding crops – especially when used carefully on genitals, better if my legs are secured apart. A warm-up is essential, starting gently and working up. Seeing a sexy video first may help (although it may set up unrealistic expectations on either side). Subdued lighting is an absolute must – candlelight is particularly good, especially night-lights inside holders which diffuse the light. The little electric flame bulbs one can buy, put inside a bedside lamp, are also good – they give a subtle, flickering, orange glow. Occasionally either one of us might wish to conceal our faces – either with masks, blindfold, or even just hiding beneath a pillow or cover – this is especially useful when working on genitals. We use 'verbals' a bit – generally he with me, calling me 'sexbitch', etc. Counting the number of strikes is also exciting, and usually my master gives more strikes than he says he will, or repeats the series if I have 'misbehaved' as a recipient during their execution.

Initially we had to build up trust. My master was far more experienced than I was. On my first meeting with him in the privacy of his own home I told him directly of my limits – no piercing of the skin, no knives. In the beginning the CP sessions were rather too severe and caused much bruising. Gradually these evolved to gentler sessions and a greater emphasis on more 'normal' sex as an outcome. I was so nervous to begin with that I set up a check system with another male friend to phone me and make sure I was okay after each visit to the master. Now we have a very satisfactory sex life together, but it took about ten years to learn what worked best between us.

Is there greater understanding? Yes, on the side of physical pleasuring and anticipating each other's moods and levels. Despite a tremendous amount of communicating, trial and error approaches and experiments, we still do not understand each other completely. Perhaps that is part of the magic that keeps our relationship fresh and alive – there are always unknown areas to explore.

If the 'top' is a man then he can support your buttocks while you wrap your legs around him and use your bindings as an additional support. It *is* trickier if the 'top' is a woman, but a firm hold round his neck and decent thigh muscles are really all it takes. And the fact that he is totally helpless makes the whole exercise deliciously exciting.

The lucky bondage devotees have ceiling beams; if not then doorways or ceiling hooks are the answer (make sure you find a joist – lumps of falling plaster are *never* very sexy). And, of course, when the hooks are not 'in use', then hanging a pot plant or a decoration from it will avoid the possibility of awkward questions.

A bed with posts is an opportunity for the classic 'spread-eagle' – a comfortable, more supported but still sexy position. Again, it leaves the 'bottom' wonderfully exposed, whether face-up or face-down and has advantages in being both maintainable almost interminably and also easily variable. If your bed has no posts then longer ties will be necessary as they will have to be anchored around the bed legs.

One thought, if using your bed for this position – consider your bed linen. A girlish pastel cover with floral sprig pattern may be fresh and lovely in summer sun, but has absolutely no erotic appeal. Dark, rich colours are what you need (deep crimson is *very* sexy) and they are flattering to every flesh tone that might end up stretched across them. Soft fabrics that slip and flow are much more sensual for writhing on than crispy cotton. So, ideally have a separate set of bedclothes to use for 'play nights'. At the very least find an erotic bedspread to use.

Another fun position to try is the 'slave girl'. Here the 'bottom' kneels and has their hands tied to their ankles behind their back. Again, this is nicely comfortable for the 'bottom', but really quite vulnerable. If a bolster or pillow is placed under the bottom and over the calves then the pelvis will be thrust a little forward – offering the clitoris (or penis, for that matter) to be played with and teased at the whim of the 'top'.

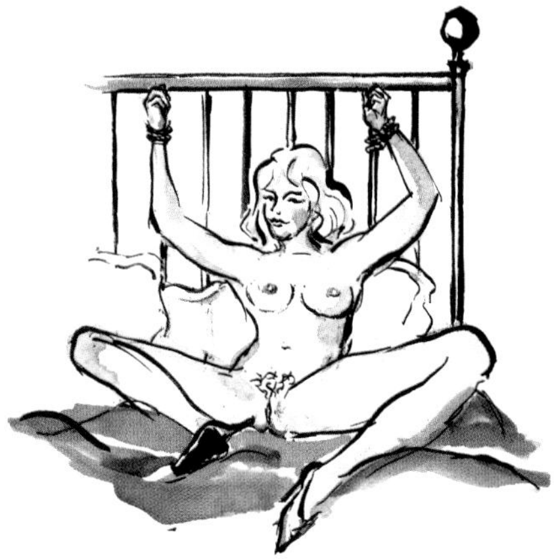

The ideal bed for bondage

One of the fun things in bondage is finding your own favourite positions. The human body can be seen as the biggest and best sex toy on the face of the earth, but do bear in mind that, unlike a toy, it does have its limits and, in bondage, you need to find what those limits of bending and stretching and turning and twisting are.

CAREFULLY DOES IT

And that is one of the main caveats – remember that the 'bottom' may be remaining in one position for some time. So the position must be tenable without any painful repercussions. Positions that require suspending the 'bottom' or even placing him or her on a chair or block need to be approached with care. Creating a 'slave auction', by placing your bound slave on a plinth for examination by prospective masters, is a great scenario to play out, but be careful with the height and stability of your plinth. This particular fantasy's bubble could be severely pricked if the whole edifice collapses.

You also need to think about circulation – positions where the arms are held above the head, or where the 'bottom' is upside down will have quite an effect on the circulation – so 'tops' need to check every so often that all is still well. And remember that the bonds must not be tied too tightly, and must come undone easily. This can take a little practice and is one of the advantages of using leather cuffs as opposed to rope or even scarves. Most certainly any bonds around the neck must be considered very carefully and should only be applied by someone who really knows what they are doing. If you are using gags it should be after negotiation – gags can be anything from a light bar to a whole ball that fits right inside the mouth and can cause restriction of breathing. So the type of gag you use and the duration for which it is worn need to be agreed beforehand.

With all the games you will play and enjoy the 'top' needs to take responsibility as well as 'power'. He or she needs to watch the 'bottom' for signs of distress or discomfort.

And as time goes on, the 'top' will learn the skill of pushing the game to its limits to allow both partners to get the maximum thrill from it without physical or psychological damage.

DUNGEONS

There's a theory that the origins of the word 'dungeon' came from the Mediaeval Latin, meaning 'The Master's Keep'. The ideal of a dank underground chamber in some storm-swept castle, hewn from the very rock upon which the stronghold was built, and from which no escape was possible, is one of dark romance. Here the bound heroine of the piece would languish, utterly at the mercy of her 'Lord' until she submitted to his wicked desires, or was rescued by her knight in shining armour.

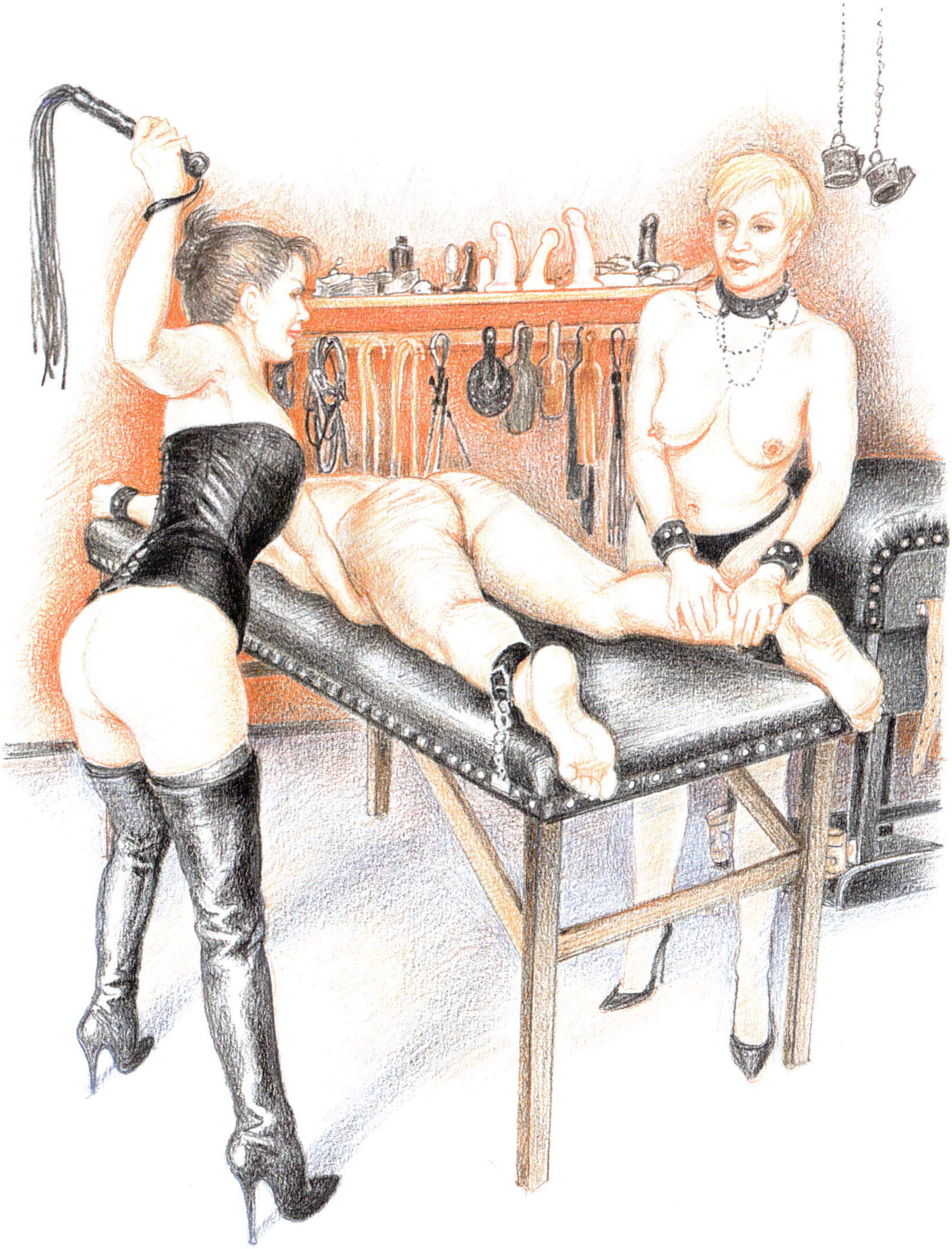

Your own personal
dungeon

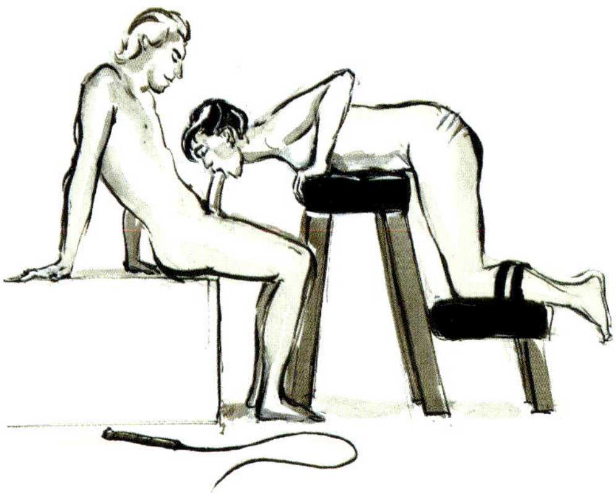

A Whipping Stool

To recreate this mediaeval fantasy in number 25 Acacia Avenue sounds like rather a tall order: but as 'dungeon play' is one of the most enduring flights of S/M imagination, there is much available to help you achieve just this. There are now suppliers of 'dungeon equipment' both in this country and abroad who will supply everything from a 'Quickie Kit', incorporating items that are easily assimilable in the general clutter of any household to 'The Dungeon-In-A-Box®'. If you're off a DIY disposition, you could always investigate the hook and screw-eye department of your local hardware store, but most items of custom-built dungeon hardware have safety features built in, so the extra expense is usually worth it. Larger pieces of furniture can sometimes be disguised so that when the vicar drops in for tea, parking his or her bottom on the very object of concealment, he or she will blissfully unaware of what sort of sinfulness has been performed upon it.

Establish which room you wish to use; usually a spare bedroom is best and preferably one situated well away from your neighbours' side of the house: the sound of whips landing on naked flesh can be very carrying, not to mention the squeals and gasps that accompany them. Most dungeons have dark walls, minimising the glow from the discreet wall lights (gels can be used to create exactly the right effect) and all sources of daylight must be shut out: strip-lights (unless ultra-violet) are not recommended. There are probably one or two larger items that no self-respecting dungeon should be without but these should be carefully chosen from a long list of imaginative instruments and pieces of dungeon furniture. These are: whipping stools, bondage chairs, gynaecological chairs, spanking horses, cages (suspendable gibbet cage, tall cage, head cage, etc.), St Andrew's Crosses, stocks and pillories, the list goes on, and I haven't even addressed the panic snaps, the double-D clips or the hog-tie clips. On the whole those who are into bondage or S/M prefer elaborate equipment and theatrical ambience.

The spanking fellowship, however, are happier to incorporate existing household objects and furniture. Ordinary dining chairs and sofas provide plenty of opportunities for bending over, kneeling on or lying across, and the naked hand or a simple plastic ruler can serve as chastising implement. Discuss with your partner which direction you would like to take and which is most practical given your domestic limitations.

For more information on Dungeons and making your own, see the index at the back for useful contacts.

FETISH AND FASHION

Firstly, don't let the word fetish put you off – it merely refers to sexual gratification linked to a particular object, part of the body or activity. So if your partner has ever cradled your foot in his hands and kissed it – if you have ever frolicked, Fergie-like, with a toe-sucker – then congratulations! You have dipped that sucked toe into the rippling waters of foot fetish. And talking of feet and fetish, let's begin with shoes.

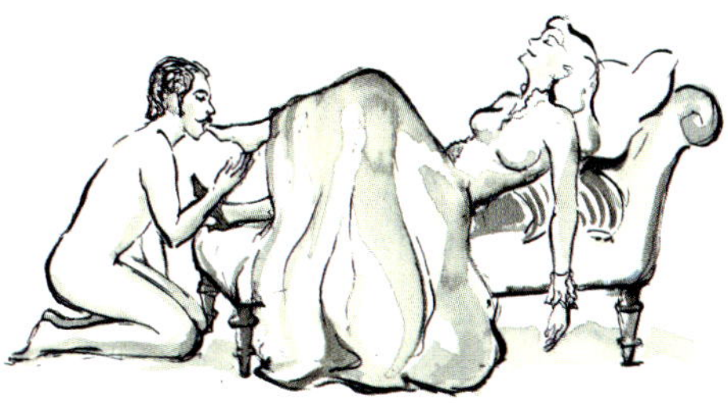

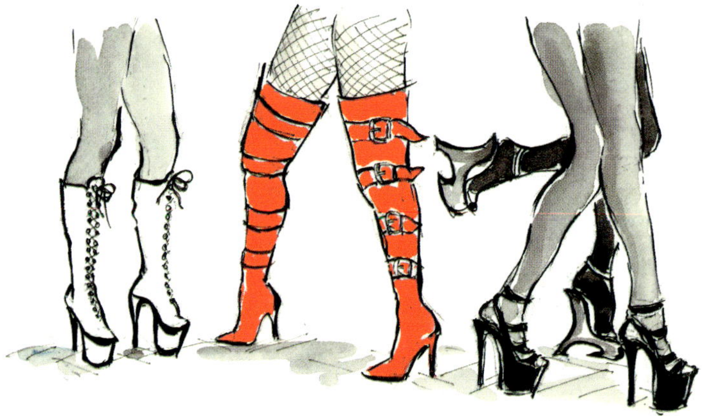

HEDONISTS IN HEELS

The classic fetish footwear is obviously the stiletto – and size *does* matter here because with stilettos the higher the better. The technical name for an accentuated appreciation of these glorious things is *altocalciphilia*. It is thought that we have Catherine de Medici to thank for the introduction of the stiletto. She was very small and, when she came to France from Italy, brought with her special shoes designed to increase her height. She started a fashion amongst aristocratic ladies which spread. And there is no denying that breathtakingly precipitous, gleaming black stilettos give many a huge sexual thrill. They're sexy for the wearer because of what they do to the rest of your body: they accentuate the curve of your spine, make buttocks and calves seem more rounded, thrust your breasts forward and give a compelling sway to your hips. They make you feel and look more of a woman. A very sexy woman. Such is the erotic capability of the stiletto that it can have this effect even when the wearer is a man – as we'll see. More usually, the erotic effect of the stiletto is appreciated by men from outside the shoe, rather than inside.

Some dominant men find that the attraction is 'bound up', if you'll excuse the pun, with the way in which the stiletto-wearing woman is, in effect, 'hobbled'. She is forced to take little steps and her helplessness along with her femininity is accentuated. Effectively she is made a fragile 'prey' for the predatory male. However, men who are 'bottoms' love the lethal appearance of the shoe, and it's men like this who frequently enjoy a little 'shoe play'. The woman needs to be balanced and supported and then she can play with the heel and the pointed toe of the shoe against her partner's naked body. Using the toe or heel around the genitals can be much appreciated – but be very careful – go slowly and watch your partner to see his response. Play around the nipples can be sexy for a man, basically using the heel as if it were a finger with a pointed nail. If the woman is seated on a high stool she can place her whole foot on the man and exert a little pressure. Once again, considerable care needs to be taken as a great deal of damage can be done with a stiletto. But – as so often – a great deal of pleasure can be had as well.

There are, of course, more 'fetishy' forms of footwear: specialist boots with sexy ties and straps, boots with rings designed to receive hooks and clips so that your legs can be held together or apart, chained to a frame or bound to your own arms or neck and, of course, superb, tight, thigh-hugging boots. These shiny, glamorous things are intensely erotic for a man to look at and touch, even kiss and lick, which, combined with the physically enjoyable stretching, elongating effect on a woman's body, is also erotic for her. And these days much of this sort of footwear is available on the High Street – as much fashion as it is fetish.

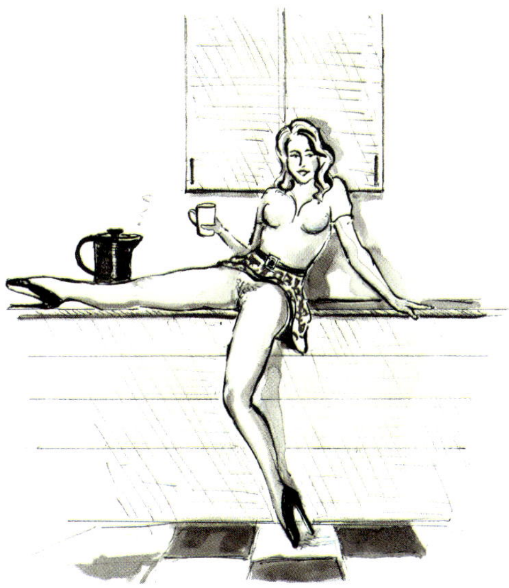

Shoes that inhibit walking

Of course, should you wish to take things a little further there are shoes that inhibit walking – shoes with impossibly high heels that leave just the toe-tip touching the ground, shoes that hobble a girl. Here we are getting into deeper waters and really bringing domination and submission into play. These shoes and boots are to be found in specialist shops and, of course, on the Internet. They are the ultimate in fashion as a form of bondage.

Before we make our way south – anatomically speaking – I would just like to point out that everything above can equally apply where it is the man who wants to wear the stilettos. Everything I said about men and bondage – the arousing effect of physical limitation – allowing a woman the 'strength' in a sexual situation – all of this applies when a man wears fetish footwear. *His* pelvis is thrust forward, *his* movement is restricted, balance is altered, steps are smaller. A bisexual friend of mine tells me that a young Adonis, waxed and in stilettos, has been in her Sexual Top Ten ever since Saxone shoe shops started doing size 10s!

STOCKINGS

Moving up the body, let's think about stockings. A cliché, yes, but they work. And they work partly because they are a cliché. When a woman puts on a pair of silky stockings, the soft flesh of her inner thighs offers itself where the lace top ends, the taut lines of the suspenders frame her front and behind and the effect is instantaneous: she begins to feel like a sexual creature. It's almost impossible to overestimate the power of lingerie.

But before we leave stockings, hold-ups are also good and come into their own under rubber or tight PVC where suspenders can create unsightly bumps. And if you don't get on with hold-ups (and many don't) then the design of crotchless tights is getting better and sexier all the time.

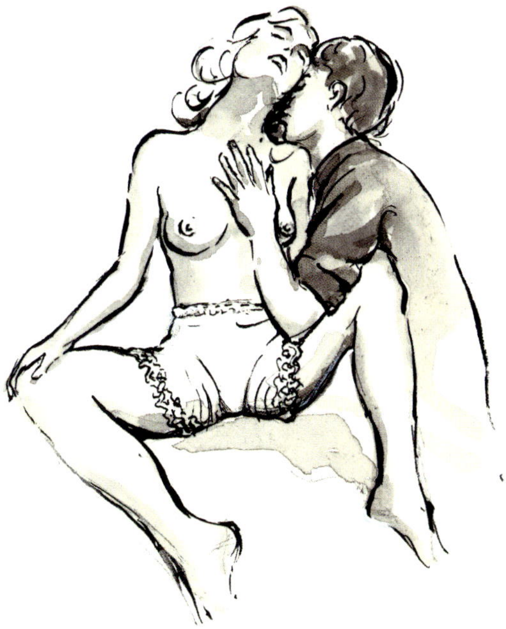

French Knickers

PANTIES

Assuming you know what they are and what they do, let's move straight on to the finer details, such as *fabric*, which can be a turn-on in many ways. A friend of mine has a lover who always wants to find her the same way: he arrives at her flat and the door is open for him. She is face down on her bed, eyes closed. She wears nothing but white ankle socks, and crisp, white, cotton panties. He says he likes the innocence of white cotton panties, the way they look, the way they feel and the way they smell. Which just goes to show that the loveliness of lingerie is in the eye of the beholder.

But, more generally, silky and slippery is good and lacy is naughty for what you can see through it and because of its delicacy. Silk is a fabulous fabric in the bedroom and what is more, it flatters a woman at the same time as feeling good. Satin is sensual, too, although a little more 'heavy duty', and great if you are going for the vamp approach.

Although materials like latex, rubber and PVC can give a frisson, be aware that they can also give a sweat rash – so be sure to try them out beforehand.

And work out where you stand on the talc front – a very good friend of mine tried out her sexy, new, rubber briefs one summer night: she shaved and talc-ed – and ended up with a crotchful of pasty white lumps. In fact, if you have a tendency to sweat then I would advise that you avoid rubber underwear.

Colour, too, is important. Think about whether this is an evening of sin and seduction or a little afternoon delight, think about your skin tone and think about what you want to say. White is that innocence again (pink too), black is powerful, sophisticated and knowing. Red is, well, a bit upfront. Explore different colours and find out what effect they have on your partner: purple, for instance is a wonderful 'end of the evening' colour set off well by a log fire, a thick pile rug and a decanter of port.

Most importantly, try to avoid wearing anything that will leave a mark. Nasty red weals bearing the imprint of elastic (even if it is as used by lingerie leaders Agent Provocateur) are never sexy. Personally, I love French knickers, partly because they are subtly sensual and can come across as either sophisticated or demure depending on the wearer, partly because they fall so flatteringly about the hips. French knickers in silk are easy to wear, easy to remove and – if you want to prolong the delight – can conceal a tiny pair of briefs or a sexy G-string beneath.

CORSETS

If what you like is something a little more *fitted* then why not try a corset.

Few things make a woman feel and look as provocative as a well-fitted corset. If she has curves, a corset will make the very most of them; if she hasn't, then a corset will give her some. It will take in her waist while it pushes up her breasts and straightens her stance. A good corset is a

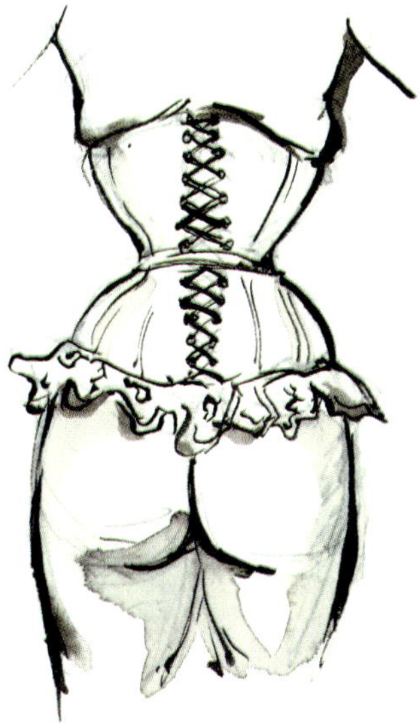

A full corset, properly laced up

fantastic feat of engineering disguised as a froth of lingerie. Some people love to wear corsets as part of fetish play. A very tight corset will not only alter body shape (eventually altering it permanently) but will restrict breathing. Both men and women use corsets for this kind of play and find this arousing. If it is an area you would like to explore then you need a very expertly fitted corset that you can lace tighter and tighter each time. But go carefully since too severe use of corsets can actually displace organs. Don't forget that the hourglass Edwardian fashion was replaced by the flat-chested 1920s fashion on grounds of health as much as anything else. If you are wearing corsets for the look and the feel then you have a great choice.

There is the full corset that goes from breasts to hips. This is a very sexy piece of 'costume' underwear and will flatter any figure. The real thing will be fitted to you by experts, like Rigby and Peller, and quite possibly will change your life. It takes some getting into (and out of) and just as long to get used to. They lace up the back and give you the kind of body

to an outfit to give a hint of fetish or naughtiness to an ensemble.

Rubber is particularly good for spanking scenes and whipping. For the Dominant who is spanking, he or she has a lovely feel – that second skin – under his or her hand. And the noise of the spank (or the paddle if one is being used) is still as satisfying. For the Submissive who is being beaten, rubber affords less of bruising without compromising the sting!

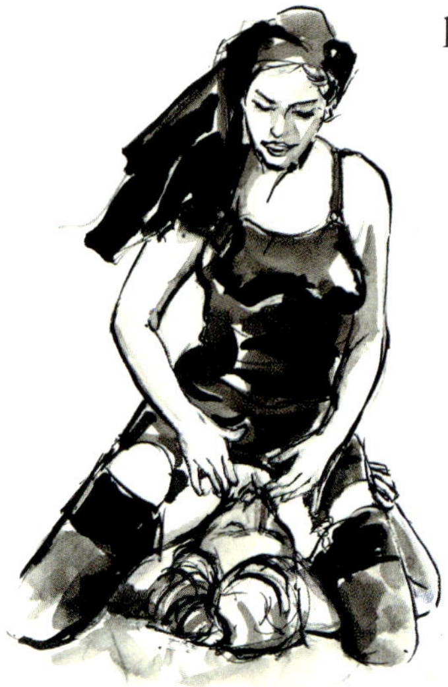

Be sure to buy decent quality rubber or it will not last. A decent gauge, or thickness, of rubber is needed for it to keep its shape during and after wearing. And check the seams: seams need to be properly overstitched and sealed. They will be coming under a lot of pressure. And it needs looking after, so when in storage keep it dry and hanging free, lightly dusted to stop it from sticking to itself. One of the many wonderful things about rubber is that a rub-down with a damp J-cloth will sort out any stains and a dry cloth with one of the glossing sprays (some people use Mr Sheen!) – that can be bought in any store where the clothes are sold – will buff you up to perfection. Rubber for sheets and upholstery can be sexy too. Just don't let it get dried out or stick to itself. And be careful with heels and fingernails.

PVC (polyvinylchloride)

Almost everything that goes for rubber goes for PVC. And PVC doesn't have the characteristic smell. It also allows for a little 'breathing' so is not such a problem for sweatiness as rubber. There are some wonderful PVC items around now; a pioneering French company makes clothes in PVC fabric which has a four way stretch built into it – it's almost like wearing

i

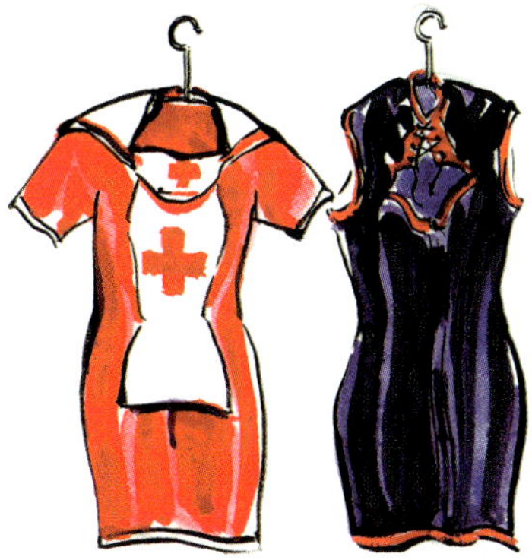

PVC Outfits

Lycra. Again, you can dip your toe in the waters by accessorising in PVC: belts and long-line gloves, collars and cuffs, boots and sexy black stilettos all add a sense of 'promise' to an outfit.

LEATHER

The look that is worth a thousand words – natural, animal, strong and very sexy. Soft leather is not the cheapest of fabrics, but worth every penny. And there's so much choice available in leather, too. As with the others, quality is all. Hard, low-quality hides may eventually break down and soften so shop with your fingertips as well as your eyes.

Dresses and skirts are very sexy in leather; bras and shorts can give a girl a sort of cavegirl attraction, too. And as for men, who doesn't fall for a man in leather? Trousers and long-line coats are tops with me: that 'Men in Black' meet the Mafiosi look just oozes testosterone. Leather also feels good against the skin, smells wonderful and gives no problems with sweat. Just don't forget that skirts, dresses and trousers can sag and bag with wear. But, on the other hand, accessories don't: wide leather belts, gloves, collars and cuffs, masks and hoods are things to look for.

Moreover, bed covers, sofas, cushions, benches and racks all have so much more of that essential 'kink' factor when in leather. Just remember that cleaning them can be a specialist business and while we like it when the memories linger on, the stains are a wholly different matter. But some things are just worth it. A single friend of mine recently bought a butter-coloured suede bed cover. He says he cannot keep women off it – there's something about its soft sensuality that encourages people to spread-eagle themselves over it and writhe around, he confides. Sounds good to me!

FUR

Fur: the ultimate luxury for some, but please bear in mind the sensibilities of animal lovers. Not everyone wants to have sex on the remains of a dead animal. But if you can't resist the sheer visceral sensation – almost the barbarity – of fucking on fur (I suppose it's that 'cavegirl' mentality again), remember, really good 'faux fur' is great, too. Obviously the plus points are the hedonistic delight of it all, the soft sensation of it on your body and the fact that a fur bedspread or rug could transform the floor of even a Butlins chalet into the ultimate love nest. The only negative point is really the cleaning: not the most romantic reason for wearing a condom – but a good one, nevertheless.

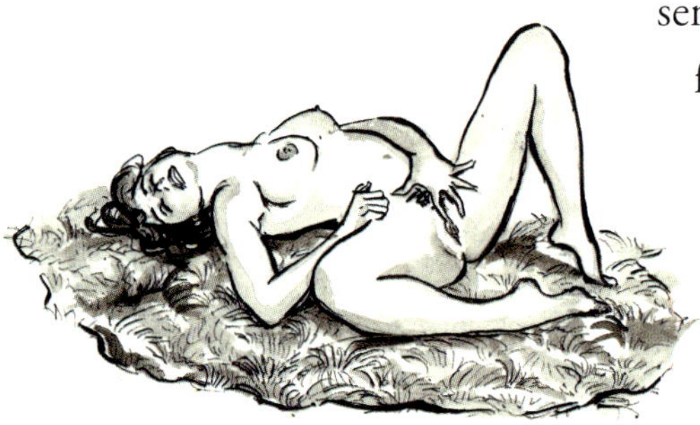

PIERCING

Piercing is all the rage nowadays. Even Harrison Ford has had his ear pierced. Be sure to go to a truly reputable practitioner who has good equipment, high standards of hygiene and who knows exactly what he or she is doing. And another piece of advice: ask someone who has had it done to them, preferably a close friend, how it feels for them. They might be able to tell you of drawbacks that you haven't considered. Almost any part of the body can be pierced. For 'sexcitement' purposes though, the piercings that are most popular are:

WOMEN

- Nipple piercing is done for decoration, for attachment of hooks during bondage sessions and (although it doesn't work for everyone) for increased sensitivity.
- Tongue piercing is said to add greatly to a girl's ability to give a great blowjob.
- Clitoral piercing (some piercings go through the hood, others through the clitoris itself) is said by some people to enhance the sexual experience. Call me old-fashioned but I don't see how it can and it sounds a bit risky to me. Some men report that they do like

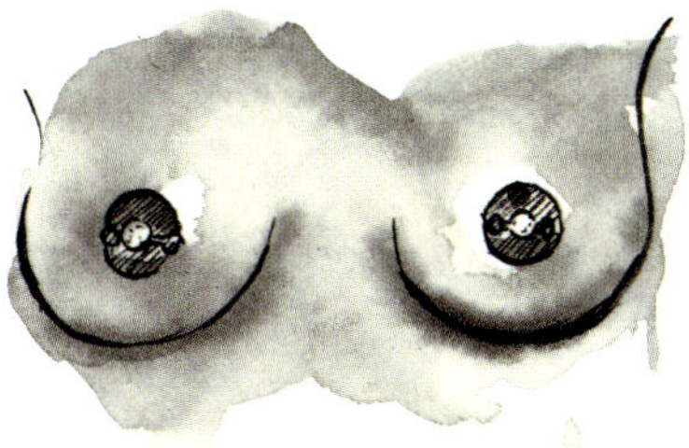

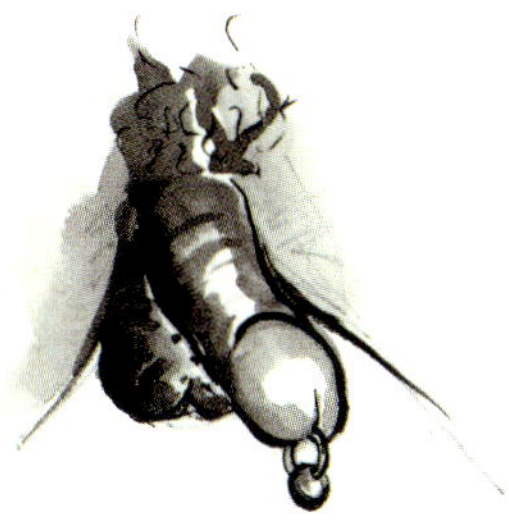

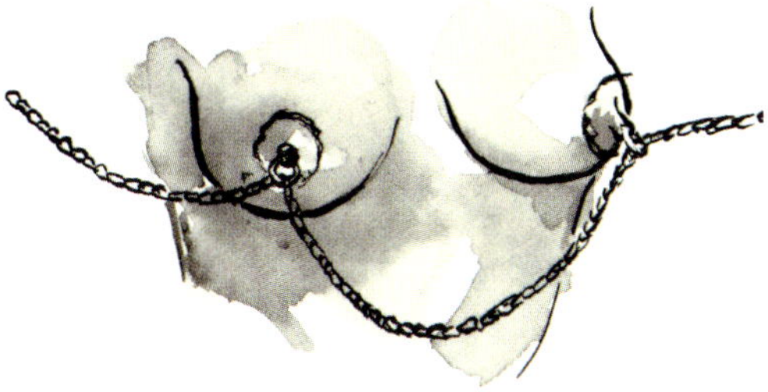

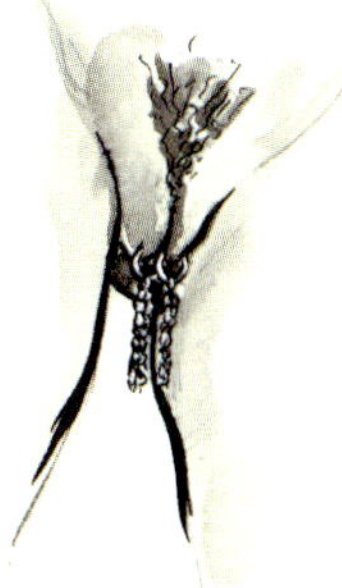

the feeling of the little ball that sits on top of the piercing rubbing up and down the shaft of their penis.

- Labial piercings are popular with those who like SM play and can have leads and chains attached like nipple piercings.

MEN

- Nipple Piercing : as above.
- Tongue Piercing : allegedly does for a boy's cunnilingus skills what it does for a girl's ability to fellate.
- Genital Piercing: There are all manner of piercings – through the scrotum and through the head of the penis itself. Once again claims are made for increased sensitivity and a colleague of mine tells me that the little metal sphere that sits under the head of his penis has transformed his girlfriend's enjoyment of sex.

Just remember that all piercings need to be maintained hygienically – especially the genital ones.

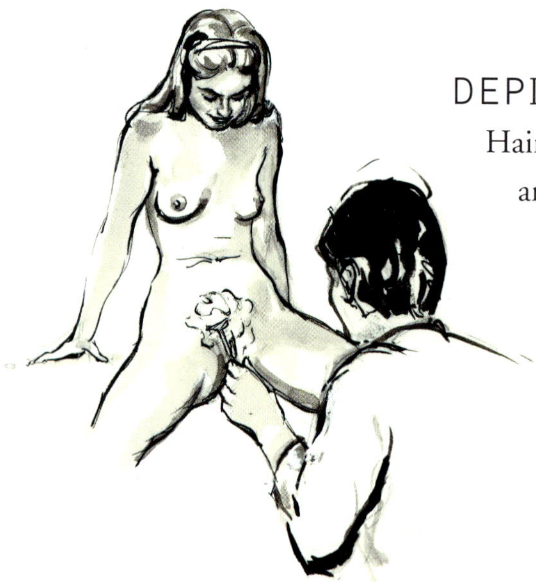

DEPILATION

Hairy or smooth is a very personal preference, and personally I have always been very attached to my 'short and curlies'. My legs are smooth and my armpits are hair-free zones, but my pubes have always been out and proud. Until a few years ago that is, when I decided that the shaven look complemented the beautiful leather corset I had just been given. In some ways the transformation was wonderful – much, much more sensitive – but aesthetically speaking, and from a visual point of view, I'm not convinced. But if you do decide to go in for depilation the choices are many these days: razor, waxing, electrolysis, sugaring, even laser – and salons are generally happy to treat men as well as women. Increasingly, some men find that they, too, like the hairless look on themselves Asking around, I was given various different reasons: "it feels better" and "I love the feeling of being licked on my bald balls" or "it is so much more sensitive, sometimes I get turned on just by the rubbing action of my Calvins" and, most frankly of all "I like to be hair free – it makes me look bigger". Increasing numbers of men are waxing all over. Chest, back, tummy and even toes are becoming top target areas for boys and their wax strips. Many women enjoy waxing their men, finding it an intimate, fun experience. Depilation can even be part of sex play. There is a real sexual charge to be enjoyed as a submissive partner, bound, helpless, legs apart while your 'Dom' wets and lathers and shaves you. It's a good game!

The only downside to depilation is the maintenance since, especially if you choose the razor method, you need to keep back the re-growth. Stubble is really not very erotic at all.

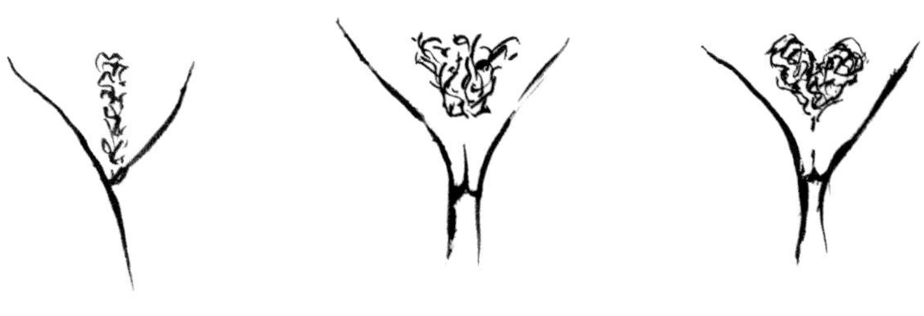

3

indulging each other

Visiting a Sex Shop Together
Toys, Gadgets, Videos and Books
Dressing Up
Photography
Awaydays
Alfresco Sex
Secret Pleasures Shared

Interview with Kathryn, one of the founders of 'Sh! Women's Emporium'

Paula What were your objectives when you started the 'Sh!' shop?

Kathryn The idea for 'Sh!' was sown a decade ago when a group of us waltzed into Soho hoping to satisfy our curiosity and have some fun. Sadly it wasn't to be. Horror-struck, we found ourselves skulking around sleaze-pits while men-in-macs leered from behind the pages of greasy mags; after all, the only sort of women they'd ever seen inside a sex-shop was the inflatable sort.

Stunned, we reeled home. Here we were, thriving in a supposedly girl-powered, guilt-free age of erotic enlightenment. Wasn't it 50 years since Dr Grafenburg had discovered our G-Spots, 30 years since we'd taken control of our fertility, 20 years of queer campaigning? Why on earth wasn't there some cosy place for women to shop for good quality, erotic playthings without feeling awkward, unwelcome or embarrassed?

Two months later, on April 1st 1992 'Sh!' was born. Our name (pronounced 'shush') is mischievous and ironic: a playful comment on how women's sexuality continues to be hushed-up. With a scanty £700 worth of stock and a large tin of pink paint adorning its walls, 'Sh!' Women's Erotic Emporium opened her doors to a trickle of appreciative women.

We're often congratulated for identifying a 'gap in the market', but this pigeonholes us, as well as crediting us with more business sense than the shop or we deserve.

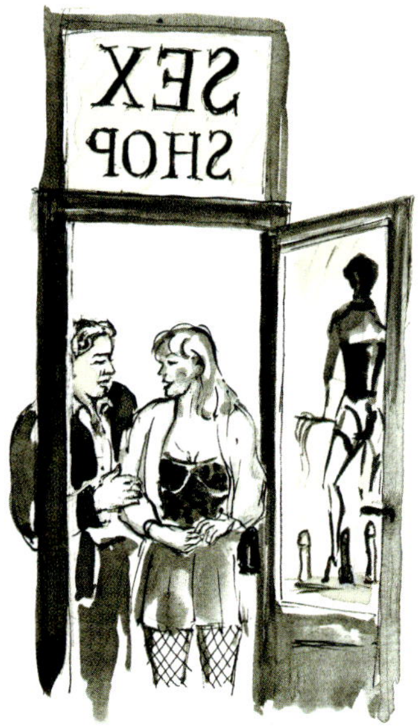

VISITING A SEX SHOP TOGETHER

I am delighted to say that the days when sex shops were frequented only by furtive gentlemen in macs who glided around Soho like grey ghosts, enveloped in a veil of anonymity, are now well and truly gone. Whenever I think of those earlier days I can't help remembering a hilarious scene from a play by Graham Greene that I saw years ago, where a couple of visitors are admitted into the vestibule of a most respectable house and see an elderly woman emerging from a loo. They go up to her and introduce themselves, only to be cut dead and ignored. The woman just walks past them and disappears into the sitting room. When the guests are shown in the old lady greets them as politely as if she had only just set eyes on them. The mystery is later explained and it transpires that the lady never acknowledges anyone who happens to espy her coming out of 'you-know-where'. How could she? According to her, she never goes to the lavatory!

This is how many men viewed their visits to a sex shop and if by any chance their wives got wind of it they could expect to be greeted at the door by a deranged Nora Batty, her bosom heaving with self-righteous indignation, wielding a formidable rolling pin. 'Visiting dens of filth and sleaze? You men, you only think of one thing!' And somehow, the men must have believed it, for they never sought to close this gaping divide between the genders.

Years later, women did begin to admit to an interest in erotic undies and sex toys, which meant that they allowed it to be inferred that they were

Yes, 'Sh!' is run very effectively as a business, but her roots are firmly planted in a passion to redress the unjust imbalance of how human sexuality is accepted in our world, with women drawing the distinctly shorter straw! There are still precious few positive role models of overtly sexual and happy women for us to look to – even Madonna has reverted to her namesake! Masturbation for women is still viewed as a sad alternative to the 'real thing', whereas for men, it's more of a case of a natural release for their uncontrollable and boundless sexuality. As women, we're told we have no taste for explicit imagery (preferring distinctly more feminine touchy-feely 'erotica'!). Girls are still branded as 'sluts' in the playground, postmenopausal women regarded as 'dried up'. Such a minefield of negative influences! Add to this the fact that women have more complex sexual responses than men and that we mature sexually later and it's small wonder that 'Sh!' – a place where women can explore their sexuality without pressure or judgement – is booming!

As 'Sh!''s birth in the early 90s coincided with images of icebergs crashing ominously through TV screens, forecasting the dire consequences of a new sexually transmitted disease, AIDS and safer-sex information always has been a priority for us. Ten years on, instances of STDs amongst young women are dramatically on the increase, so empowering women with information and self-knowledge remains top of our list.

P Did you find at first that women were reticent to set foot inside?

K The big difference between 'Sh!' and other apparently 'women-friendly' stores is that men are welcome to browse only when accompanied by a woman. This means no single woman will come through our doors and be outnumbered by blokes – it is her domain. Nor will she be bombarded by graphic magazines, nasty 'realistic' toys, naff blow-up sheep or scary zip-mouth hoods because we don't sell these. She'll be offered coffee, and given all the help, advice – or space – that she needs. Much of the 'Sh!' experience is passed by word of mouth and certainly lots of women skip into the shop proudly. But centuries of negativity around female sexuality have worked their influence on all of us (send me into a newsagent for a top shelf mag and watch me squirm and make excuses that 'it's for work'!) and certainly all through 'Sh!'s life, women have obviously made two trips around the block before working up the courage to come through our doors. Even though we're working hard to put right the imbalance, ten years in the context of centuries is not going to reverse that.

P How many couples visit the shop? What is the age range?

K Lots of couples come to 'Sh!', especially on Saturdays. Men seem to enjoy the comfortable atmosphere where they can ask questions without being branded 'dirty old men'. The age range is refreshingly wide – from eighteen to eighty.

P Are people willing to discuss what they are looking for with the

masturbating regularly, and they even acknowledged leafing through a top shelf magazine occasionally if they found it left lying around. There began to appear the erotic equivalent of Tupperware parties where girls could sit gossiping and giggling while they examined the latest in vibrators and crotchless knickers. This was all very fine, but that still meant that the sexes were separated. Why, oh why, couldn't men and women at last get together on this matter, since they were both inevitably dependant on each other when it came to doing it?

Part of the problem was that most people tended to see sex shops as catering only for 'wankers'. It was assumed that the items they sold would not be necessary if you had a fulfilling relationship, and no one considered that toys and aids and erotic books might enhance a relationship.

At last we are beginning to see sex magazines (such as *Desire*) that cater for couples. They have a totally different feel to them. At last women can pick them up and read informative, helpful articles, many of them actually written *by* women, about real sex. By contrast, in the typical old-style 'girlie mag', women provided the embellishments but never the ideas; the text was full of fast cars and over-lubricated adventures purporting to be the real-life experiences and feelings of the pouting models. None of these told men anything real about the women they live with but simply perpetuated typical male myths.

What was missing was the shop counterpart to the enlightened sex magazine. I'm pleased to say that at last they are here – woman-friendly, couple-friendly sex shops. For a full list see the appendix at the end of this book and be sure to read the interview accompanying this chapter.

TOYS, GADGETS, VIDEOS AND BOOKS

Sex toys are a growth industry. Currently there is so much to choose from that the mind reels. Whether shopping from your local sex shop, the Internet or a direct mail catalogue, the bad old days of being

assistants? Do you get much feedback about how they liked what they bought?

K There's a lot of information sharing. We've certainly learnt a good deal through our years of sex-toy selling and we pass this on in store and in our catalogue. But a sex toy is the most personal, most intimate thing one can buy and advice about how to choose is not (yet) passed on from mother to daughter. So we don't hold ourselves up as experts; after all, no toy is a guaranteed orgasm-provider and expectations, as well as claims by the manufacturers (8 inches of pulsating pleasure will have her in ecstasy all night) can be ridiculously high. Information is a two-way street in our shop and there's been many a discussion over the vibe and lube stands! All our toys are displayed so they can be touched or turned on. Women are practical shoppers and how loud a toy is, how warm it is to touch, how long it might live, is more important information to give than the exaggerated claims on the packaging. We get feedback in lovely forms – letters telling us that after seven years of marriage and three kids, a Jessica Rabbit vibrator finally gave this woman her first orgasm or that on the advice of one of our assistants, a simple bottle of lube made lovemaking sensual again for a 70-year-old couple.

But we're not starry-eyed, either. Both in store and in our catalogue, we talk about the downside of vibrators: these mass-produced 'novelties' can have unpredictable life spans. Unprecedented in this business, we offer a thirty-day guarantee on all battery-operated toys. Even so, the disappointment of women whose toy has died in 6 months upsets us almost as much as it does them and we look forward to the day when sex-toy manufacturers buck their ideas up.

P What sort of items are the most popular?

K It's no surprise that vibrators are bestsellers. A woman's complex sexual response often requires sustained stimulation of her clitoris to reach orgasm, which these relatively cheap, portable, effective little gadgets happily provide. Lots of women tell us they first reached orgasm with their handy little buzzer. Our best selling model is called 'Jessica Rabbit'. We put its popularity down to two specifically female-friendly design features – the twirling beads that stimulate the entrance to the vagina (where we're most sensitive inside) and her 'pièce de résistance' – two split bunny's ears to stimulate the sides of the clit rather than smack bang on it which many of us find too direct and intense. The effect of the 'Power of the Purse' (women having access to choose for themselves rather than those toys brought home by their bloke from some suburban 'private' shop) is making manufacturers more inventive in their designs and we're now able to offer more clit-specific toys. It's taken years, but designers are finally conceding that size actually isn't everything and that women will often use a vibrator solely to stimulate their clitorises.

Strap-ons come in a close second to vibes in the popularity stakes. In response to the unimaginative and

limited to one overpriced choice of vibrator, inflatable doll, dull condom or tacky, badly made piece of lingerie are no more than a distant and vaguely unpleasant memory. These days you're more likely to be handed your purchase in a shopping bag complete with a smart logo and a bright 'Thank you for shopping at…' than slipped a brown paper bag with a knowing smirk. Having said that, there's always room for improvement and of the high street chain stores, Harmony seems to be getting it most right. Their interiors are spacious, well-lit, and their staff friendly; there's a genuinely unisex shopping atmosphere and (usually) a good mix of different types and sexes – just as there might be at your local

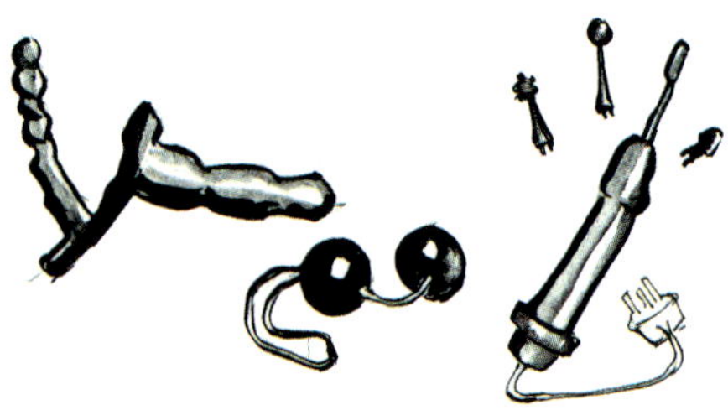

supermarket. Talking of which, a little shopping around before you buy could be advisable: at the time of going to press another retail sex shop chain was charging way over the odds for a tube of lubricant that you could buy at Boots for a *far* more attractive price.

Most sex toys and gadgets are fairly self-explanatory, but their novelty is always entertaining. A great deal of fun comes from the 'how the hell do we make this work?' or 'this is outrageous, the manufacturers can't *seriously* expect us to…' reaction. (For an utterly hilarious and anarchic look at the sex-toy industry try The Erotic Print Society's *The Illustrated Book of Sex Gadgets.*) On the other hand, it may just be a case of replacing last year's model; like a serious cook going out to buy the raw materials or essential equipment for a sumptuous banquet, you could know just what you need. You will be looking for exactly the right ingredients – and nothing less will do.

Commercial sex or porn videos are certainly not everyone's idea of mutual arousal. There is a general move afoot

impractical models offered by wholesalers we decided to manufacture our own designs. Our harnesses come in soft, easy-to-wear leather and our dildos come in a colourful array of over 40 sizes and styles. The majority of strap-ons are sold to lesbian couples from all over the world (such is their fame!), but an increasing amount are now sold to straight couples (probably about 30%) for women to pleasure the prostates of their men – a phenomenon that warms the cockles of our hearts.

P Would you say that there are more women today who are happy to explore their bi-sexuality and talk openly about it?

K Many recent influences – stores like ours, where women can feel free to explore their sexuality, the 'Sex and the City' girls, the 'sexualisation' of 'lipstick lesbians', most programmes on Channel 5, the drug ecstasy, the outlawing of homophobia – all seem to be breaking down taboos around girl-love. Lesbian and bisexual women are definitely coming out and openly expressing and identifying themselves without fear of ridicule or attack. Happily this millennium seems to be the one where the limits labels are bunged in the bin where they belong.

P Could you mention some new gadgets or toys that we may not be familiar with?

K We've been hearing from our friends the doctors and nurses at St Mary's sexual health clinic of new products from the States that are mini clit pumps – devices designed to vacuum blood into the clit, to engorge it, creating heightened sensitivity and we'll definitely be getting stocks ASAP! New toys are being made in a material called 'cyber-skin', a lovely product that feels velvety and peachy to touch. We're also hearing from HIV professionals that 'Nonoxyl 9', a detergent sometimes found in lubes and once thought to be a possible HIV virus-killer, is actually a very dodgy product whose harshness can actually make transmission routes easier so we're spreading the word about that, too.

P Kathryn, thank you. I can only add that when I visited 'Sh!', it certainly made me feel that I was in a more erotic atmosphere, and it was really helpful to be able to discuss the items with friendly women assistants.

to make porn more palatable for sharing couples, which is to be lauded, but this book is about the sexual excitement and sensual experiences that you can generate with your partner by using your *own* imaginations, not the voyeuristic dross churned out by a huge, cynical industry that's often repetitive and, quite honestly, rather dull. Of course there are 'specialist' fetish movies that may be essential partner viewing if you are both going in a certain fetish direction. There are also some (very few, sadly) erotic movies on video that *are* made by directors with flair and sophistication – Tanya Hyde, for example. But with the wonderful digital video cameras and equipment now available why not make your own 'amateur' porn video? After all, your great-grandchildren

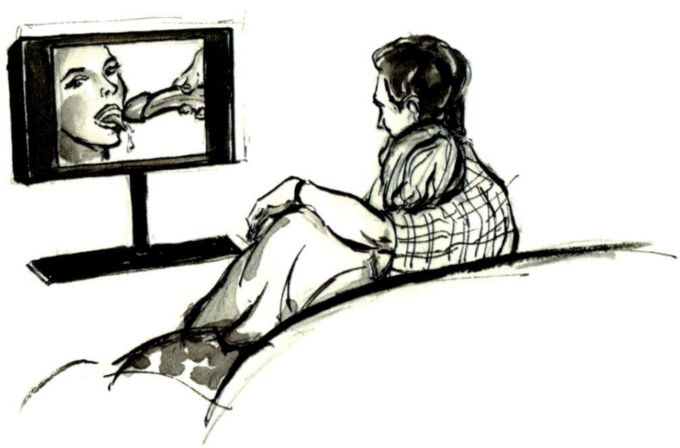

will need *something* to remember you by…

Reading bits of erotic fiction to each other can be a marvellous aphrodisiac. Try something from The Scarlet Library's range of classic erotic fiction. Or perhaps your tastes will run to something more contemporary. It's my experience that men find women reading explicit passages to them in a low, husky, sexy voice almost irresistible. I wonder why. Perhaps it's somehow the same as 'talking dirty' – only with style. Become the ultimate Edwardian maidservant or decadent aristocrat by selecting certain passages to read – or even enact – together. Many bookshops have an erotica section and if you are reading this book you're probably well acquainted with the Erotic Print Society's backlist.

Whatever your tastes or requirements, the best place for information on these fun items or crucial accessories will come from the appendix giving details of retail outlets, websites and direct mail firms at the end of this book. Happy shopping!

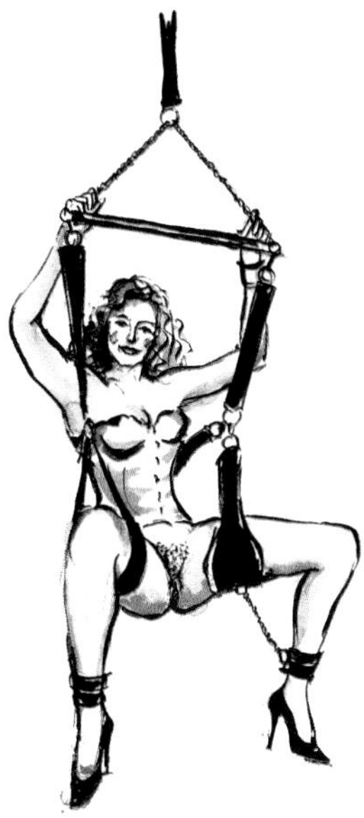

A love swing is obtainable from specialist retail outlets

DRESSING UP

When you live with someone you probably see them slopping around the house dressed in ordinary, comfortable clothes, or smart but unimaginative ones for work and there may not be many occasions when dressing up to look and feel sexy is appropriate.

Nowadays it is not thought very politically correct to dress up for a partner, especially not for a woman to do so, but this notion is just an understandable backlash from the days when females were seen too often as passive sex objects. We really don't need to be touchy about dressing up for each other now. How about a little more of the active sex *subject*?

It is true that sexy clothes tend not to be the most comfortable, but that is for a purpose; it is to draw attention to our erotic attributes. When I am all kitted out for a party, the last thing I feel is comfortable. As I described earlier, the high-heeled shoes thrust your body forward, exaggerating breasts and nipples, the tight dress makes you aware of holding your tummy in, and your bottom seems to have expanded lewdly. Special bras create cleavage, and thongs slightly tug between the buttocks while suspenders pull every time you sit down, but, regardless of all that, personally, I usually feel *wonderful*. It's only much later, when tiredness starts to kick in, that all these clothes are stripped off with relief and cast aside.

Dressing up just to please your partner is one-sided. It's much better if you enjoy it too and revel in the effect you are having. I agree that it's mainly women who are expected to put on a show but that's because they usually carry it off better and there are a lot more choices for them in the female wardrobe. All the same, I think men could experiment a bit more with underwear. When you are sitting down at a restaurant table it's exciting to remember that your companion is wearing a sexy black leather jock strap, or transparent flimsy briefs, just as he will be thrilled to know that you are not wearing *anything*.

In the privacy of our homes we can build up a wardrobe of favourite costumes. I believe there could well be an exhibitionist lurking in most of us and if that exhibitionist can be coaxed out he or she could be the key to helping us free ourselves from inhibitions. Another word from Lucy Bailey:

By dressing up in a costume you are actually helping to set the scene. They help you take on a role, not just physically, but in how they can make you feel. Some costumes make you feel powerful, while others make you vulnerable. Being fully clothed or completely naked are quite different states. When you are naked you are exposed and unprotected, it can be humiliating especially if those around you are clothed. It is interesting how wearing a certain costume changes your personality. I think this is because you lose your inhibitions and sense of self. Possibly the costumes we choose are something of an 'alter ego' within ourselves. When I put on a school uniform I immediately turn into a wild St Trinian's girl, having immense fun being naughty. I start misbehaving by provoking and irritating the people around me. Something about that uniform makes me feel childish and irresponsible. In most scenes, whether they are playing the submissive or the dominant role, it is the women who end up dressing the part. You love seeing her all dressed up, say, in seamed stockings, high heels and a tight blue nurse's uniform. Have you ever considered that she might want to see you as a New York Cop or leather clad pirate? I think it's about time men started making more of an effort to dress appropriately for scenes.

Uniforms seem to be the attire most popular for CP scenes. This is probably because of their past associations with the institutions of school discipline and judicial CP. Uniforms are an instant symbol of your social status, either indicating that you hold a position of responsibility or the opposite. Part of the scene can involve the submissive being inspected for their 'turn out'. The dominant will check for smartness and make sure that all items are regulation. Punishment can then be dished out adoringly for any infringements. I must admit that I find men in uniforms very sexy. I suppose it's because they look so powerful. My favourites are a Naval Captain's uniform and a British Army Parade uniform.

Lucy also mentions wet spankings where the sub has just got out of the bath or a swimming pool, or you can just make them wear wet knickers. 'Bottoms always look so delicious with wet clinging pants/panties adorning them,' she says. Here's an idea for the non-spankers too. It's not for nothing that 'Bollywood' films frequently feature young women in wet saris. Wet, clinging muslin is very sexy, especially when your nipples are erect and standing out underneath it! Have you ever tried clingfilm? Get your partner to wrap it tightly round your body and you will feel as sinuous as a snake.

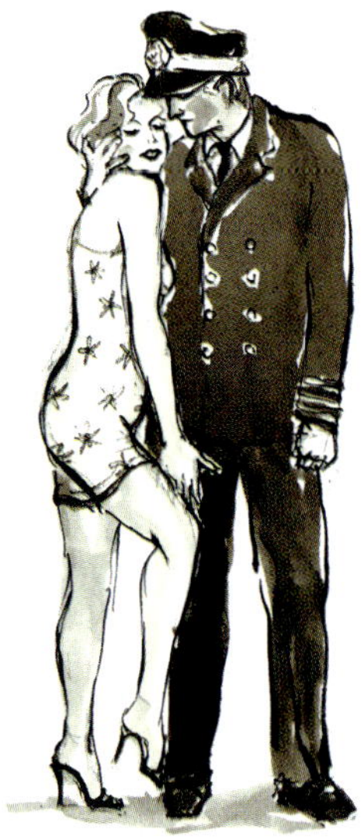

Whether it is fetish wear or more theatrical costume, dressing up is an excellent encouragement, and when you add in a camera, only the most seriously repressed could fail to respond. Of course, not everyone is necessarily quite such an incurable exhibitionist as I am, but if you've ever had occasion to don a costume and perform on stage you will be aware of the effect it can have on your personality. I remember how different I felt playing a Victorian maid in a TV costume drama when I had to wear a corset and an enormous hooped skirt, which swung around and took a lot of controlling. One had to walk *so* demurely to remain decent. The sensation of wearing those clothes was remarkable: from the waist up I was all pinched in, and from the waist down it felt as if I were completely naked. The white starched cap and apron completed the picture of submission and I immediately became one of the invisible classes who knew that nothing they had to say was of the slightest importance to their masters. I cast my eyes demurely downwards and found that this state felt mysteriously sexy. At any minute I could find myself upended and ravished in the laundry cupboard… Nowadays our fantasy maid would be a lot more foxy and naughty, with her ridiculously short, black, shiny dress showing frilly suspenders under its hem whenever she bends over to put down her tray of drinks.

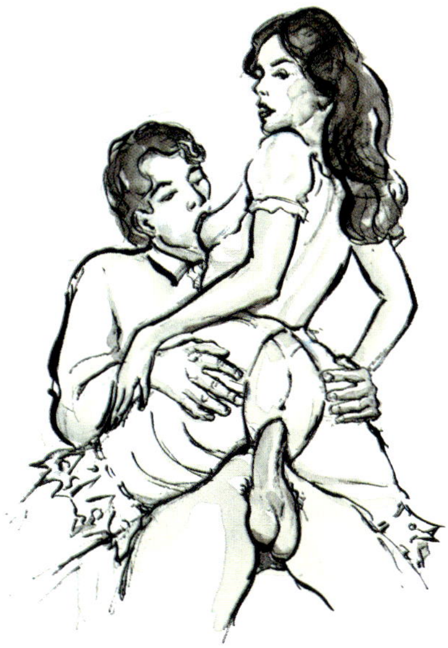

PHOTOGRAPHY

As I suggested earlier, why not make your own videos? All right – they may only have 'amateur' status, but they are still great fun to watch. Plan your own scenario loosely and set the camera up to cover the area you intend to use. Stick some masking tape on the carpet as a guide to prevent you from going out of shot. You will get a better result if you invest in some lighting; two light sources are better than one. Although your video is not going to be of broadcast standard, it will be frustrating if you can't see what is going on. Try to remember not to block the action. If you are filming a scene where you are spanking your misbehaving little maid, try to make sure you do not stand between her bottom and the camera. Try to stand her at an angle to the camera so that both her facial expression and her buttocks are visible – there is nothing more boring than a close up on one static bit of a person's anatomy without their face reflecting the sensations they are feeling. Women with long hair need to tie it back if they are going to be effective giving a blowjob; hair can obscure all her special efforts.

I'm sure I don't have to remind you to label videos clearly. Don't re-use one of your home erotica productions for recording your friend's wedding, for example; it would be most unfortunate if you were sitting down comfortably with the family watching this innocuous home movie, only to be unexpectedly confronted by huge, close-up images of your own bare bottom tacked on incongruously at the end of the tape. There would certainly be a panic-stricken search for the remote control.

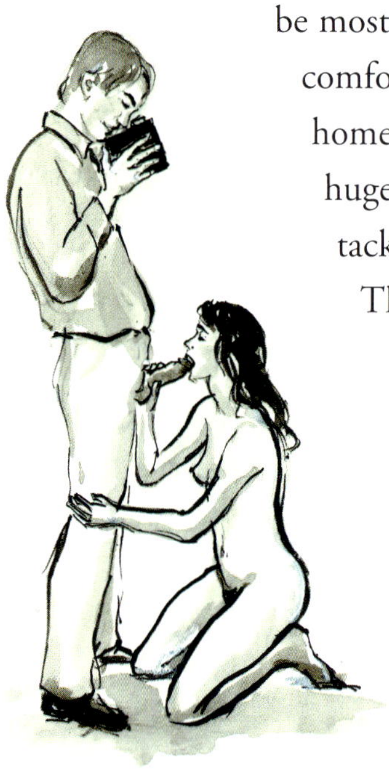

Bringing out your camera adds another dimension to the scene. The camera implies an invisible audience out there – all those who might one day see your 'performance' – even if it is only going to be you. It gives you a focal point to play to and a purpose. There are those who find the very presence of a camera enormously arousing and liberating. I must admit that I am one of them and if the photographer happened to be a boyfriend, the accumulated excitement and tension between the two of us could be put to good use afterwards. One of my favourite roles for a photo shoot was a fourteen-year-old student, all innocence and pigtails, who seduces her private 'tutor' by allowing her short skirt to ride up, flashing her naked pussy at him as she lolls inattentively at her desk. I think playing this character helped to make up for my misspent youth; when I actually was fourteen I hadn't the faintest idea about anything!

There are those who can reveal a deeply hidden side of themselves when the camera's lens is directed at them. The photographer Grace Lau makes these interesting observations about the effect of the camera on cross-dressers, in her book *Adults in Wonderland*:

The camera as catalyst is a phenomenon that I have become progressively more aware of, and acting in a cathartic role is another unexpected feature of my work… most of my clients feel sufficiently comfortable in my presence to reveal their fantasies as long as I respond to and acknowledge their masquerade. At times I feel I have become the mirror for my cross-dressing clients, reflecting back their feminine beauty, even though I am actually looking at a rough, heavily-jowled and painfully shaven masculine face with pursed over-lipsticked mouth and layered foundation. But by engaging with their masquerade, I provide the necessary assurance that they crave.

Gender reversal is a subject we will return to later. The point here is that the camera is a useful reflector, showing us aspects and expressions of ourselves we never knew we had. When you first see yourself naked, openly doing something explicitly sexual, it may be a revelation, it may

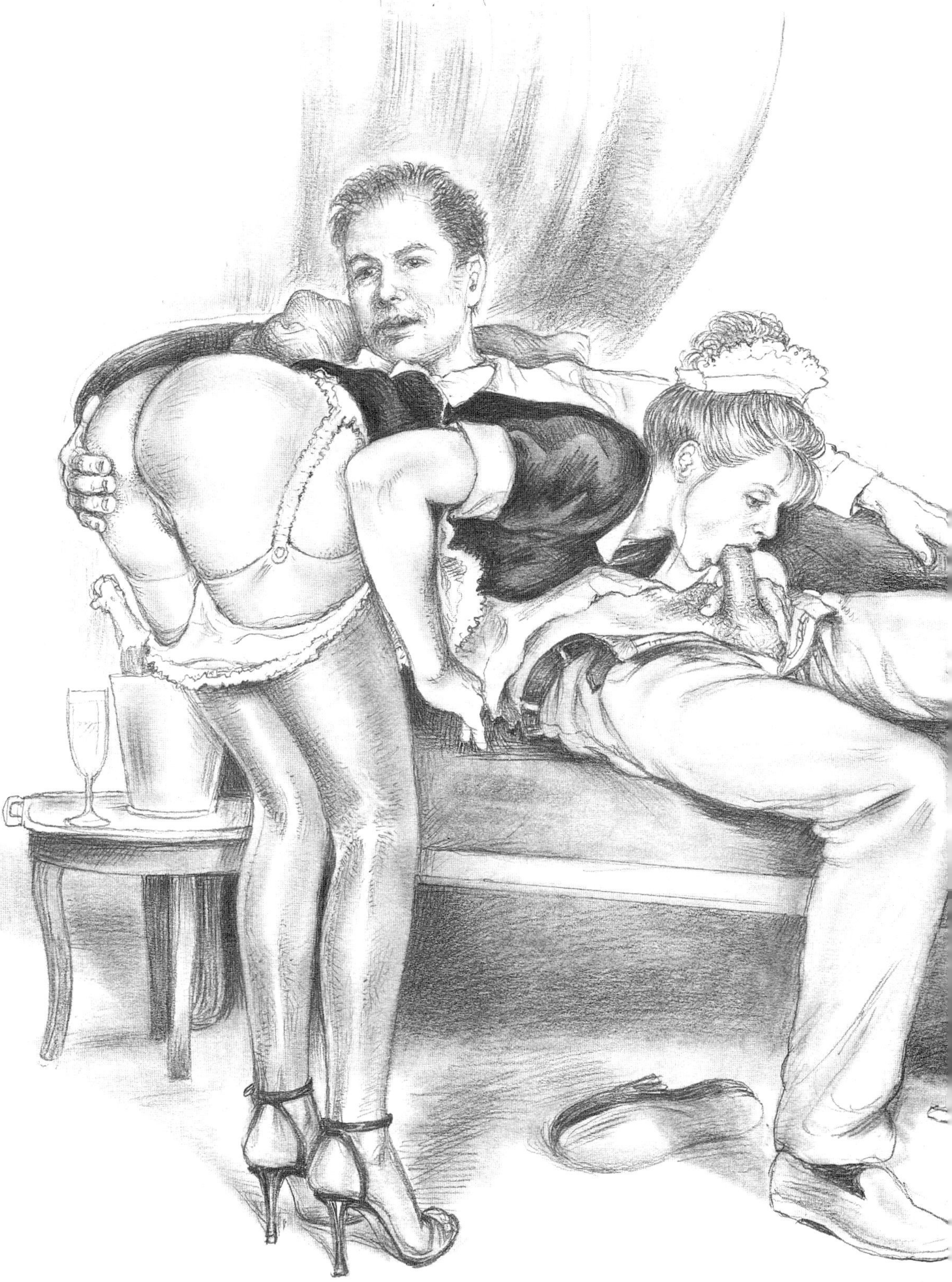

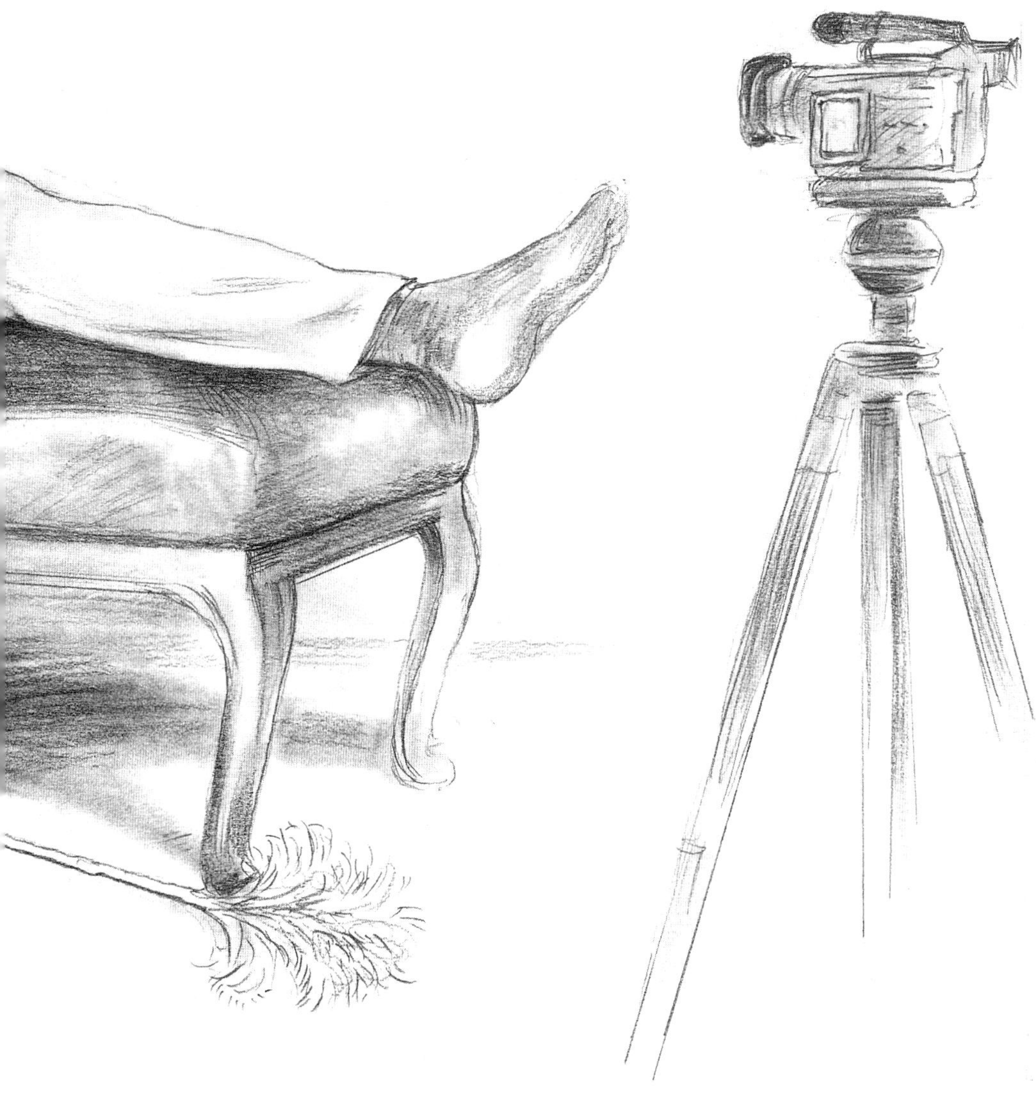

Filming your Misbehaving Maid

even be a shock, but it will help you to fully accept yourself as a sexual being.

AWAYDAYS

Do you find it hard to get into an erotic frame of mind sometimes? It happens to all of us, and if you have children it is doubly understandable. What you need is to treat yourselves to an occasional Awayday. The domestic environment is never conducive to role-play that takes time and preparation. We often fear getting decked up in our favourite corset or harness, only to hear the doorbell ring and find our sister has come round for a chat. Particularly risky is the situation where you have got yourself tied up and cannot be extricated in anything under ten minutes.

Many years back, my partner and I both had a day off work and decided to have one of our submission days. It was my turn to be dominant and I had thought it might be a good idea to try him with a little bondage. This turned out to be the first and last time we ever did it. I had my man stark naked over the living room table and had tied his wrists and ankles with rope to the table legs, taking great care that he was securely held. (Nowadays I would dissuade anyone from doing this; always make sure that the knots you tie can be easily undone!) Suddenly we heard our good friend from the flat below making his way upstairs. He tapped on the door and then opened it a chink and we froze. I think he must have seen us before the door closed again, but I heard myself informing him that we were just having a nap and I would come down and talk to him later. The dear man never referred to the incident but it was particularly awkward for my partner who felt that our friend would now regard him with an amused twinkle in the eye. It wasn't as if he even liked being tied up, and he never wanted to be placed in that position again (literally).

Now if this had happened when we were away, staying in a hotel, and it had been me in the compromising position, the result would have been quite different. If a handsome young waiter delivering room service had tapped politely on the door, just at that very moment when I had been secured to the bedposts with naked bottom thrust expectantly in the air, he would probably have been admitted. For if it is a good hotel, the well-trained factotum will behave like a veritable Jeeves, delicately averting his eyes and never making remarks. You tip him and he says, 'Thank you, sir', with impeccable grace, and withdraws as if he hadn't noticed anything untoward. The more wicked side of me would enjoy that very much.

When you are staying in a hotel always make a note of those that have useful erotic extras: a good bed-head with rungs is excellent for those with bondage proclivities, and a four-poster has similar advantages, as well as the fantasy elements. A large bath or Jacuzzi is luxurious for pampering and bathroom games.

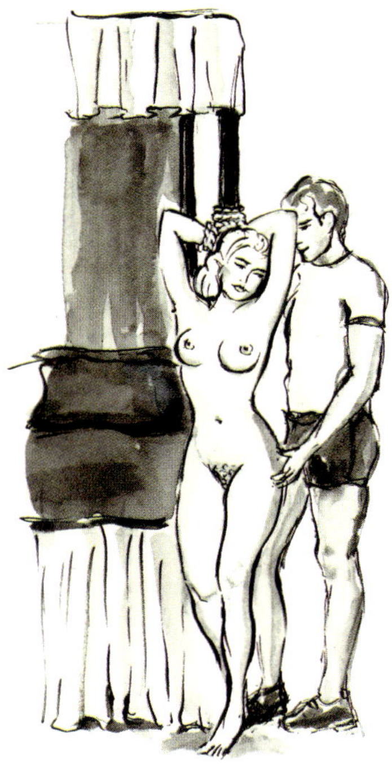

When you are in another environment it is much easier to assume a new erotic role, and maintain it for as long as you want. Developing the idea of a 'submission day' for one of you can be a wonderful relaxation. The submissive may be the one who has many decisions and responsibilities in their normal daily routine and to be kidnapped for a day of unexpected delights where everything is organised for them is just what is needed.

The hotel does not have to be plush and expensive to give us that erotic charge. Sometimes the slightly run-down, bohemian atmosphere is more romantic. For this, Paris is ideal. Who cares that the room is slightly seedy, if it looks out onto a Parisian market and the eighteenth century rooftops of that magical city; it can serve for a different kind of fantasy. You can get yourselves in the mood with a leisurely walk down the rue St Denis and then take your naughty *putain* back to the hotel room for a sleazy night of uninhibited lewdness.

Don't forget to come equipped. Obviously you don't want a lot of bondage equipment and canes to tumble out of your suitcase accidentally. I suggest you select the more convenient items of kit and buy a special small case – it need be no more than a foot long – to keep them in. Your selection of necessities could include any or all of the following: smaller silicone dildoes, harness and butt-plug, two coils of soft rope, and cuffs for ankles and wrists (with clips for attaching to rope), nipple clips, lubricant, extra tissues, short handled suede flogger or martinet and a small paddle. Don't forget you will probably already have the perfectly innocent bedroom slippers, and a battery operated toothbrush doubles up as a very effective vibrator for use on the clitoris (I refer, of course, to the non-bristly side).

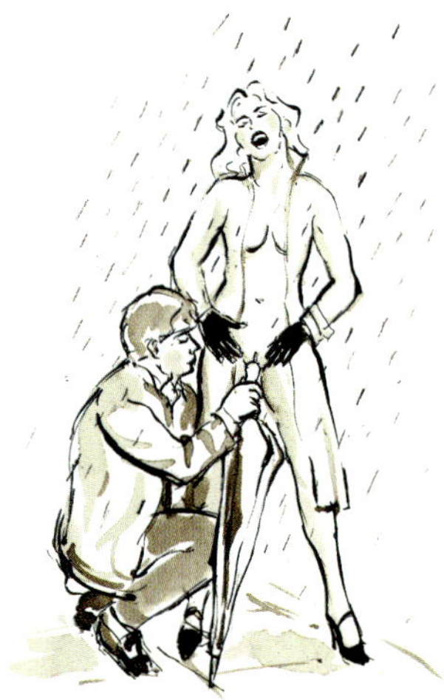

Anything can be used to pleasure yourself

You don't need me to suggest what clothes

you bring. Many women have tucked away those exotic undies given to them as birthday or Valentine presents (and never worn); well, now is the time to try them out. If you have properly prepared for your Awayday by visiting a sex shop or lingerie and corset specialist, you will already have an array of new goodies to explore. Always remember to pack several extra pairs of sheer stockings for they might well come in for a rough time, and make sure to include the digital camera for recording all the best moments. These can be printed out and mounted in a special Awayday private album. They will be your shared secret and run alongside your other holiday snaps to remind you of what you did when you weren't gazing at the more usual sights outdoors.

ALFRESCO SEX

Alfresco fucking – literally, sex outdoors (but increasingly taken to mean sex in public places) – presents a whole new range of challenges to the couple who are determined to keep their love life sparklingly fresh. Woodland, deserted parks, the moors, the heath, the hill, the mountainside, your back garden and even the potting shed in your back garden, surrounded by net curtain-twitching neighbours, are all possible 'outdoor' locations. Planes, cars, boats, trains and buses; the list is long and as long as the chances of discovery are few and the reprimand, if there is one, good-natured, then – what are you waiting for?

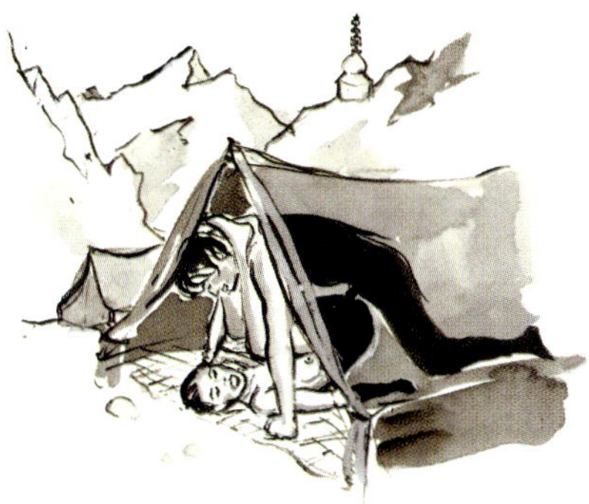

DOORWAYS

Doorways of shops are good late at

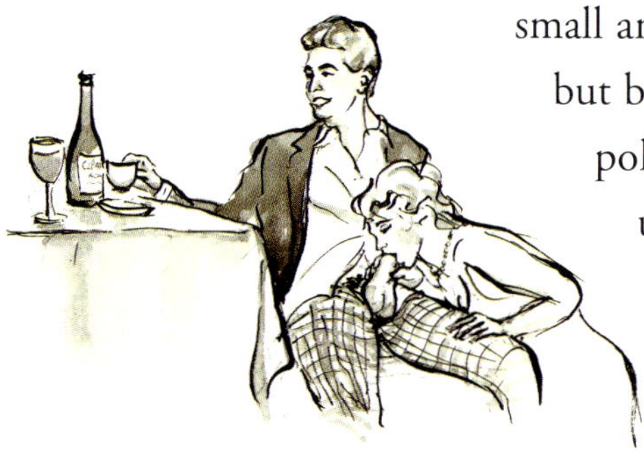

night as they are often recessed and give some small amount of cover for a knee-trembler, but be on the lookout for a patrolling police car. They might think you were up to something *far* worse.

PARTIES

Outdoor parties, barbeques, weddings or simply big cocktail parties can be boring. So why not liven things up by strolling into the garden and finding a deserted gazebo, summerhouse or even large hedge or bit of topiary to have sex in or behind? Each location will have its own peculiar charm. Watch out for brambles and nettles, inquisitive dogs with cold, wet noses with their walkers only a few yards distant and pesky insects – wasps, mosquitoes and even determined flies can be a real distraction. Also, don't forget about grass- and mud-stains. They could tell more of a tale than you bargained for when you re-enter a roomful of people. And if you're anywhere near a nature reserve, beware: recently badger-watch cameras caught a Lake District holiday couple in full alfresco fuck. Their particular brand of wildlife was transmitted to every room of the local hotel via its nature watch channel. Come to think of it *all* outdoor locations are prey to the ubiquitous CCTV, and no doubt in the near future there will be a reality TV programme devoted entirely to candidly captured cavortings… but I don't want to put you off. Sex in the great outdoors is one of the simplest and most direct ways to get back in touch with Mother Nature.

PLANES

There are obvious places and times to do it on a long haul flight, but here are some tips: plan ahead with loose-fitting clothes and leave off underwear to avoid attention-drawing squirming; and don't expect to have great sex on a crowded, London–Edinburgh business flight; a half-empty, late night, transatlantic one is what you need. The dark, in-flight movie period is a very good time, as is any time when the cabin crew are preoccupied with preparing a meal. The loo is a great place for mile-high sexual intercourse, but make sure it's not at peak traffic time: it's not easy to persuade an irate queue, hopping from foot to foot, that you were merely trying to extract a splinter from your partner's big toe. Not all aeroplane loos are designed in the same way, but they are all small, so make use of the cramped conditions to brace yourselves against unexpected turbulence and into interesting positions; the mirrors and relatively low lighting in an otherwise lavatorial atmosphere contribute to the excitement. And do remember that the cabin crew will take great pleasure in unlocking the door and whisking it wide open if they get any complaints, so obey their instructions and don't annoy other passengers by being too noisy. Back in the cabin, the female partner can discreetly sit on your lap and move herself up and down, but the most romantic position to my mind is to raise the armrest between you and throw a travelling rug over yourselves from the waist down. Then all she has to do is hitch up her skirt and turn on her side, while he just 'spoons' in behind her.

TRAINS

The same applies to trains, and if you share a sleeper, this can even invite conventional sex with the comforting, rhythmic sound of the wheels on the track.

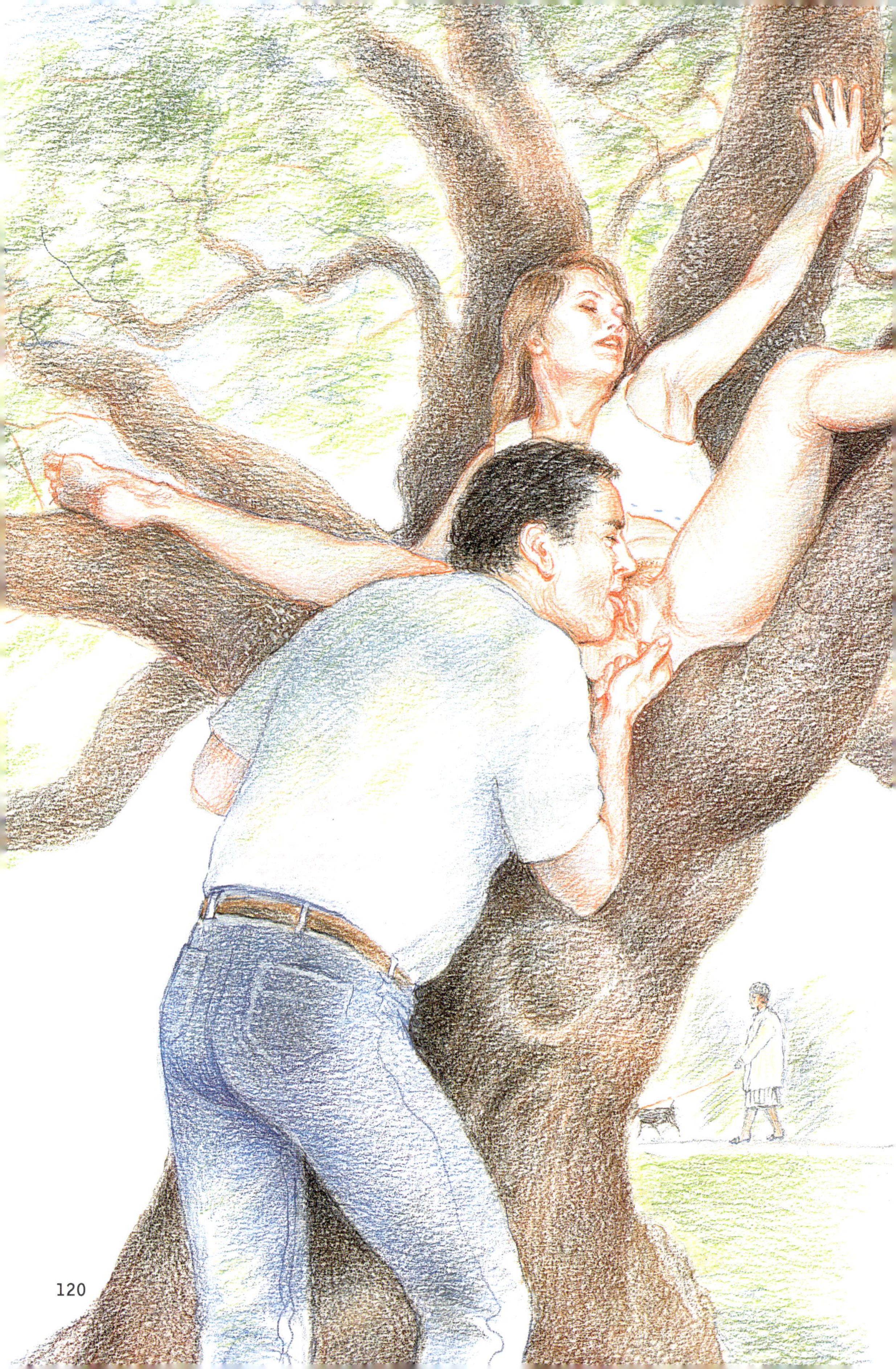

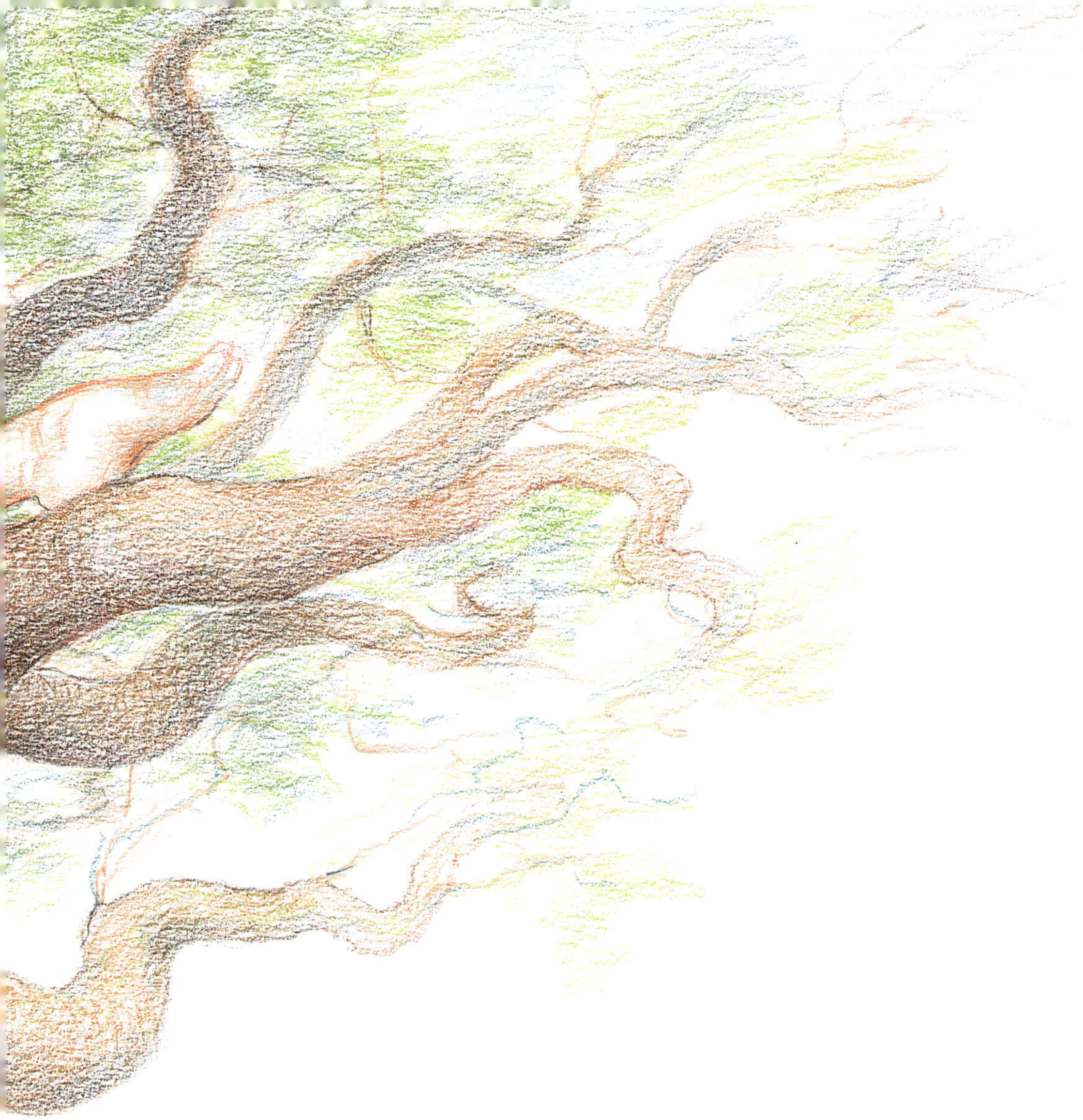

Communing with your favourite
tree can be a special turn-on

BUSES

Even more of a challenge. Put a good few empty seats between you and the other passengers. But I'm reliably told that magnificent things have been achieved on long-haul Greyhound bus journeys.

BOATS

Shirley Valentine experiences on Greek fishing boats are great – but don't come home reeking of diesel and covered in black engine oil… and watch out for sunburn.

CARS

Haven't we all done it in an old banger? Really? Well, if you're a newcomer to this game, remember that you will need impenetrably tinted windows and even then you may get a tap on the window and a supercilious 'Would you mind stepping out of the car, please Sir/Madam?' at the critical moment. Or look up to see a couple of manic 'doggers'' faces pressed up against the windscreen, contributing the sort of audience participation that you'd rather not have.

RESTAURANTS

Unless you're into toe sex under the table, it's the loos again, I'm afraid. But these aren't unisex usually, and management could take a dim view if you are caught in the wrong gender-designated toilet. You might have to leave quickly and skip your Black Forest gateau. But I do know of one couple who managed to have perfectly respectable oral sex in their local tea shoppe. The place was almost deserted; the service was abysmal and there was plenty of time and scope for a quick, but satisfying, blowjob.

EXOTIC HOLIDAYS

Another boon for the alfresco sex seeker. Some friends of mine went on a

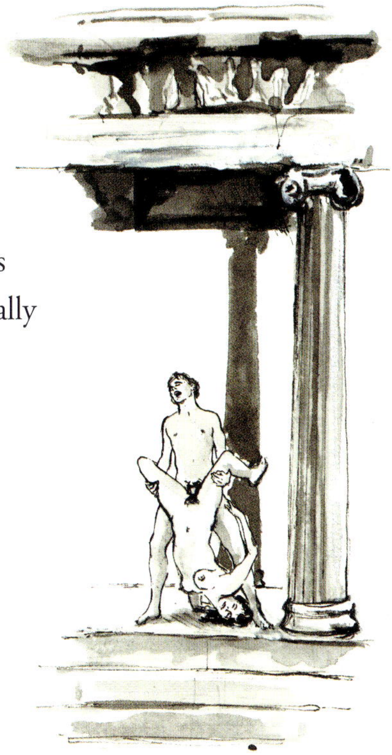

trekking holiday in the Himalayas and had blissful sex at thirteen thousand feet while their children slumbered gently in the next-door tent. Safaris at lower levels are presumably good for this sort of excitement, too. Historic locations are usually well-guarded and rightly so. But if your goal is an orgy of rampant outdoor sex rather than one of destructive vandalism, what could be more thrilling than re-enacting some primitive ritual in a prehistoric site or in the ruins of a classical temple on a balmy night under a starlit sky? If you can dodge the security staff, that is.

SECRET PLEASURES SHARED

This is a very intimate area between most couples, not unlike a 'shared joke' that excludes everyone else. Not so secret, perhaps, that you can't communicate it to others after the event, but at the time of its occurrence it is an act that is both exciting and clandestine.

Perhaps the best example of an 'SPS' is the knowledge that your female partner is sitting down to a candlelit dinner in a smart restaurant without her knickers. Or that in the same restaurant, the husband has surreptitiously undone his flies so that his partner might tease his cock into hardness by running the sole of her foot over his naked balls.

Now that sex-toy technology is becoming increasingly sophisticated, it's quite possible to go to a party, or a concert, or some other social outing, with a remote-controlled vibrator in place. If your male partner has a particularly vicious streak, he will wait until you're talking to the Secretary of your local golf club before flicking the switch. Or if he's feeling more charitable, to that tall, dark, handsome man/woman you always said you had a slight crush on…

'SPSs', like alfresco sex, come naturally to us when we are young and in love, and are part of the bonding proccss bctween couples. But there's every reason to revisit that place in a sexual relationship, where anything seemed possible, where a secret code developed as you got to know one another better and better. A certain phrase could mean 'I'm feeling impossibly randy, let's get out of here and find somewhere to fuck – *now*!' or 'I'm thinking of your cunt/cock at this very moment. It's making me incredibly wet/hard' and so on. As discussed in the 'awayday' section (p.114), getting out of your everyday environment is not just a tonic and an aphrodisiac, it's an absolute *necessity*: not only are you free of any reminders of the daily drudge, but you can also be wonderfully, creatively *anonymous*. You can be staying at a hotel and leave your room at separate times, agreeing to meet in the bar downstairs. Depending on your temperaments, one of you might want to play the mysterious, beguiling single, while your partner plays the seducer. The excitement is heightened and becomes less innocent if there are others, unaware of the plot, who try to get in on this act: it is not without a little inherent danger.

I'd like to conclude this chapter on indulging each other with this simple peice of advise from a married friend of mine in her 40s:

Don't ever take each other for granted; busy lives and tiredness should be more reason to make extra special times for each other. Instead of thinking, 'I can't be bothered, I'm too tired', think positive! 'How can we relax and enjoy each other?'

When imagination stirs, so do the emotions. The first home could set up an easy dinner and leave it on low so that it can be eaten any time, younger kids to bed, the older ones on a trip to the cinema.

Run a hot bubble bath with candlelight, glass of wine poured and ready. When your partner arrives home, sexy kisses to the back of the neck, soft talk of relaxing with a glass of wine in the bath. Lead them, gently helping them to remove their clothing, followed by more soft kisses until they sink into the bubbles. Kneel by the bath, talking softly to them as they unwind, sliding your hand under the bubbles to stroke and fondle them under the water. This is guaranteed to heighten the senses. Gently sponging bubbles over the top of their body, give them more soft kisses between sips of wine, then eventually the two of you will be in the bubbles together. Up to you where you go from there. Dry each other and lead your partner into the bedroom whatever sexy fun you wish to create followed by dinner in bed, after which you can just sink into a sleepy sexy cuddle before sleep, or the second round!

Surprising your partner with one of their talked about fantasies can really stir up very passionate responses... chocolate sauce painted onto parts of the body and licked off on a picnic, for instance; arriving to meet your partner in a public place with no knickers on and finding a semi public place where you can prove it is a wonderful turn on, even if you have to wait until later to fulfil it!

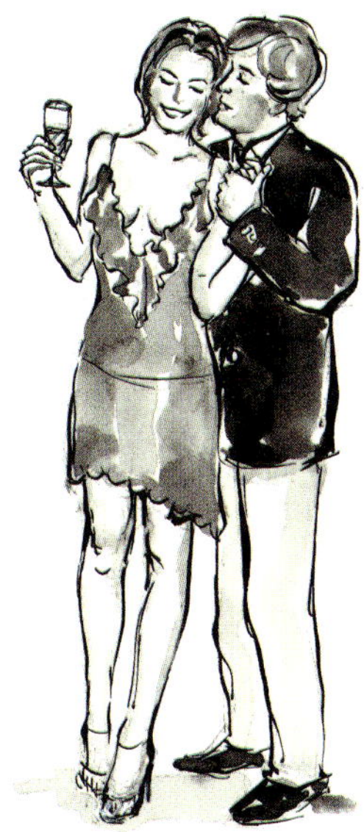

It really is seduction all over again, and again! Just open your mind and tempt each other, want each other - it will fire the passion between you. And remember, open your eyes too and look deep into your lover's eyes; then you will see the pleasure as well as feeling it.

4

is anything taboo?

Watersports
Anal Sex
Piercing and Tatooing
When Bondage Becomes Dangerous
Fisting
Dildos
Experiments with Gender Reversal

WATERSPORTS

Watersports are much more widely enjoyed than you might think. Firstly, let me emphasise that human urine, freshly expelled, is a sterile liquid. You won't catch anything from it. If you are going to explore watersports then remember the old adage 'you are what you eat'. So drink plenty of water for plenty of nice, mild, golden, pleasant-to-play-in pee. And what you do with it is up to you.

You can start gently with a little voyeurism: some men like to watch a woman pee, and vice versa. You can do this standing or crouching. A nice idea is to position the woman over a glass bowl or tank and have her pee into that, creating a great view for the man. Also, the female partner can hold his cock, 'firehosing' it while he relieves himself: this can be good, naughty fun, especially if you're outdoors. If you want to move on from that you could try a 'golden shower', where one partner lies under the other who stands. The standing partner then pees on the lying partner. The sensation is warm, intimate and actually rather nice. If wished then the other partner can return the favour. If this is happening indoors then rubber or plastic sheeting is advisable, unless you want to use a floor, a bath or a shower.

Some people like to go one step further and drink their partner's pee. This is, of course, is perfectly safe. Indeed if one takes the advise of many well-known personalities down the ages, it is positively health-giving.

ANAL SEX

I know lots of people who *love* anal sex, but it has to be appreciated that it is not for everyone. Obviously there is the question of hygiene, and this is what seems to worry people most. Generally speaking the rectum is clear of faeces and so anal sex shouldn't really be any messier than vaginal

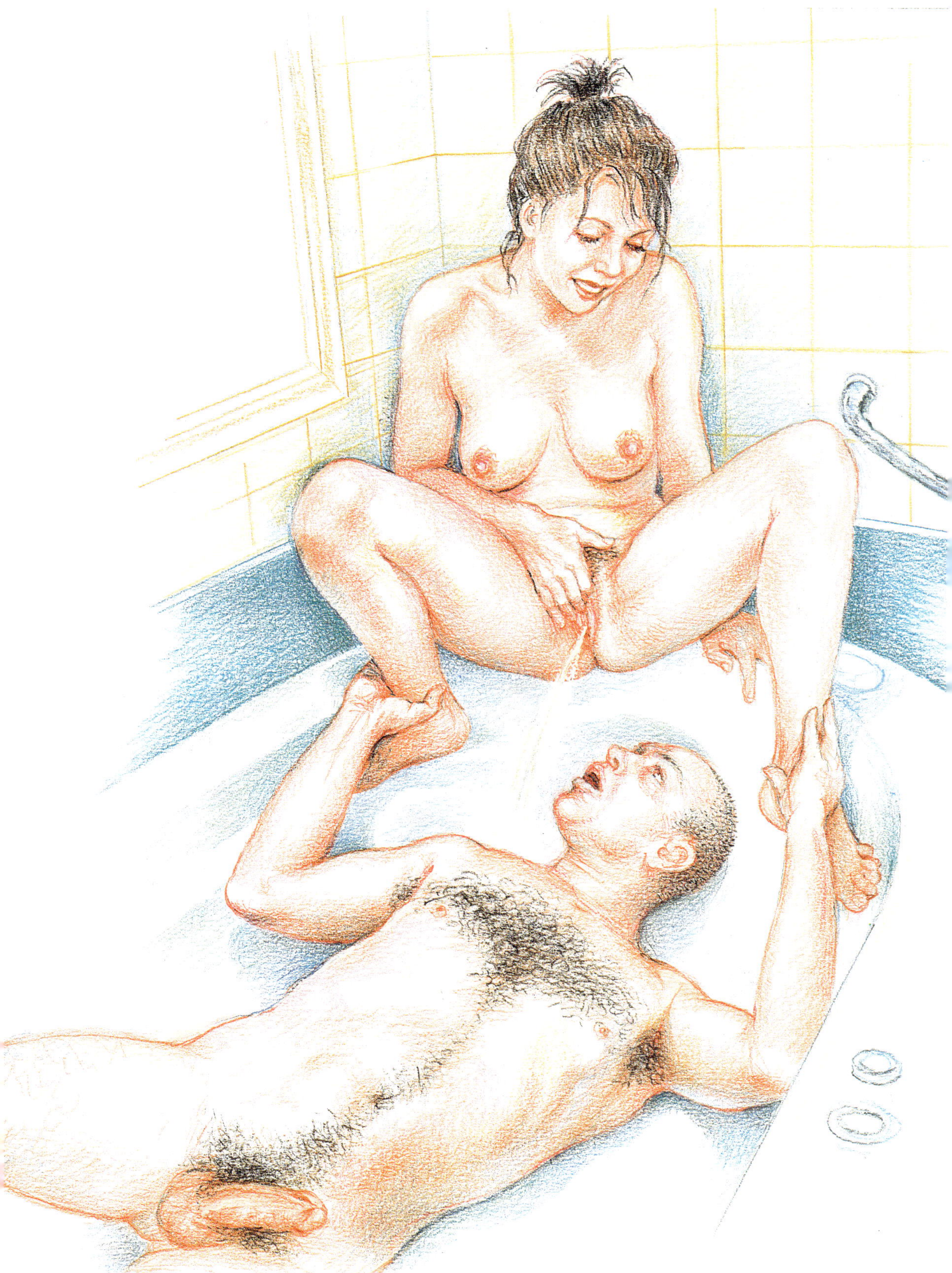

Some men like to watch a
woman pee

or oral sex. There may be the odd stray bit of faecal matter lurking sometimes, especially with deep penetration, and you both have to be OK with that. Otherwise an enema to douche the anal canal and rectum can be used before sex, but ideally you should leave at least two hours between having the enema and anal sex. Douching/enema equipment is simple to use and is available from most chemists. And remember, you can always wear a condom – it's really the least elaborate way for the man to keep his cock 'clean'.

ENEMAS

Enemas are primarily intended to clean out the rectum. They are very simple devices to introduce warm water to the rectal canal, which is then released, taking with it any detritus lurking there. However, many people like the sensation of an enema: the feeling as the water enters, the fullness and then the release. Some people like to play together, giving each other enemas, either as part of role-play or just to clear out the bowels. Enema kits are readily available, simple to use and there is an argument for trying anything once, but they should not be indulged in too often, as this tends to upset the body's normal functions.

RIMMING (ANALINGUS)

OK... so you have doubtless tried, and hopefully enjoyed, cunnilingus and fellatio.

Rimming is the art and practice of tonguing and licking around the anus. This can be wonderful to give and to receive, either on its own or as a prelude to anal sex.

Many men, in particular, find this soft, non-threatening anal

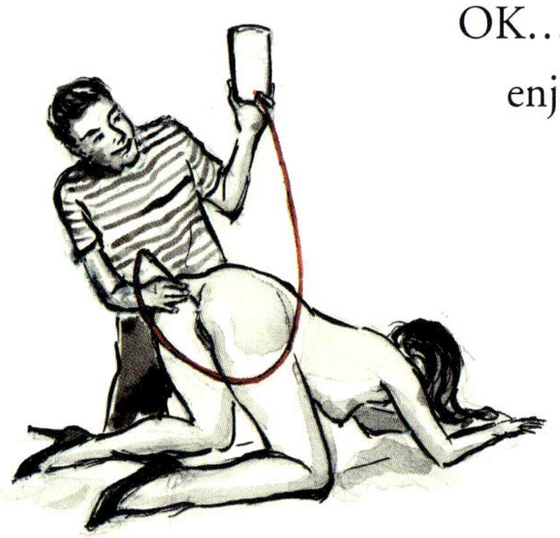

Enemas

stimulation arousing. The anus is a wonderful, nerve-rich, sexual playground, once you get past the hang-ups and taboos that surround it. You just need to be aware of the hygeine issues. The back passage is home to many kinds of bacteria and these can lead to anything from stomach upsets and yeast infections to worse. When it comes to having anal sex the man should not move his penis (or fingers) from anus to vagina, or, needless to say, mouth. It is always advisable to wash after anal sex. Having said this, thousands of long-term partners seem to practice analingus and anal sex, without any ill effects at all – just make sure that you keep this intimacy to your partner alone.

Insofar as more specifically sexual health is concerned, if you have thrown away the condoms we have to assume that you are very, very sure of each other. Which is fabulous, but remember that the tissue inside the anus is very delicate and more prone to tearing and fissures than that inside the vagina.

The tissue of the walls within the rectum allows for absorption – which is why drugs can be administered in suppository form. For this reason, infection is more easily passed on in this area of the body.

Many STDs and genito-urinary infections can remain without symptoms for years – everything from chlamydia to HIV. But if you want to be absolutely sure, tests for anything and everything are easily done and widely available these days.

With some of the more extreme practices, or with rough, hard or deep fucking, problems such as cystitis can flare up which can lead to all manner of urinary tract and kidney infections.

But don't let all this health talk put you off completely! It's really no more than common sense. And if you stopped to think about the bacterial possibilities of your every action you would seal yourself into a sterile bubble and never come out again.

HOW IT ALL WORKS

The anus has around it two very powerful rings of muscles called sphincters, one internal and one external. These muscles are not really made to relax on penetration in the same way that the vaginal muscles are. In fact they are designed to expel, not to accept. But a mixture of desire, love, patience, relaxation and lubrication will allow penetration and open up a whole new world of pleasure for both of you. As an alternative, and if your anal adventuring is being planned in advance, you can buy a few butt plugs of varying sizes and work your way up in size to something approximating your partner. You will learn to relax and gain confidence with the whole thing. Practice, as they say, makes perfect.

You should also remember that the rectum is not designed to self-lubricate, as is the vagina. So using a good water-based lubricant is an absolute *must*. I can't say I can recommend KY as it dries very quickly, but Body Glide, Wet Platinum, Liquid Silk and Probe are brilliant and remain slippery for ages. Some are great fans of saliva – although it has a fairly minimal effect and, until you are both enthusiastic and practised, it's probably not advisable. But why not have fun finding your own favourite slippery stuff?

Now, if you have decided to go for it, let's talk positions. Here you need to find your own favourites. Just like the clitoris has a slightly different configuraion in different women, and every vagina is angled its own sweet way, the rectum, too, is an individual inroad. Everyone is just a tiny bit different and that difference can make one position more or less comfortable than another.

DOGGY STYLE

This has all the benefits of vaginal doggy style sex and really, if you are new to anal sex, is by far the easiest position to start with. The woman kneels on all fours, presenting a pert and inviting arse to the man; he can take his time, is in a good position to get a good thrust and the depth of penetration is easily controllable. It enables either the woman or the man to indulge in some clitoral play, the man can play with his partner's breasts and the woman can reach back and caress her partner's balls.

STANDING

This is very simple and has all the plus points of doggy style. The penetrating party simply stands behind and bends his or her partner over a table, a sofa or… well, just use your imagination. All I will say is that however good a washing machine on spin cycle feels when you are on your own, it feels *so* much better when you are hard up against it while someone is hard up you.

THE OYSTER

The woman lies on her back with her feet over her head. Again this gives the man good access and control. It can be a little uncomfortable and you may feel very stretched, but that can be nice. A variant of this position has the woman with her feet up on the man's shoulders.

SPOONS

The couple lie on their sides, with her back to his front. This is a very relaxed, egalitarian position. The downside being that the man has much less purchase and thrust. Now the woman needs to help him by pushing back towards him.

COWGIRL

Girls on top! Gives tremendous depth of penetration and lots of control to the woman. Plus a marvellous view for the man as his partner straddles him, facing him. He can play with her breasts and clit as she rises and falls. The woman needs to make sure that the angle of her body is right and the man needs to have a really good, stiff hard-on to get the benefit of this position.

REVERSE COWGIRL

This is just the same as 'Cowgirl', only with the woman facing *away* from the man.

These are the main positions, but as always, there is so much fun to be had in finding your own variations.

After all these 'dos', just remember:

- Don't rush it.
- Don't force it or keep going, if it feels bad.
- And don't let anyone push you into having anal sex if you are anything less than intrigued by the idea. A bad experience can damage not just physically, but psychologically and emotionally, too. So go gently.

WHAT'S SAUCE FOR THE GOOSE...

The anus is a wonderfully sensitive orifice for both sexes and this means that anal penetration can be incredibly arousing for boys too. It must be remembered that anal play and, especially, penetration is something that must be approached sensitively with men (for more on this subject, see experiments with gender reversal, p.144).

DOUBLE PENETRATION (DP)

If a woman likes anal sex then she may want to progress to 'double penetration'; this can be achieved in many ways, but most simply by using

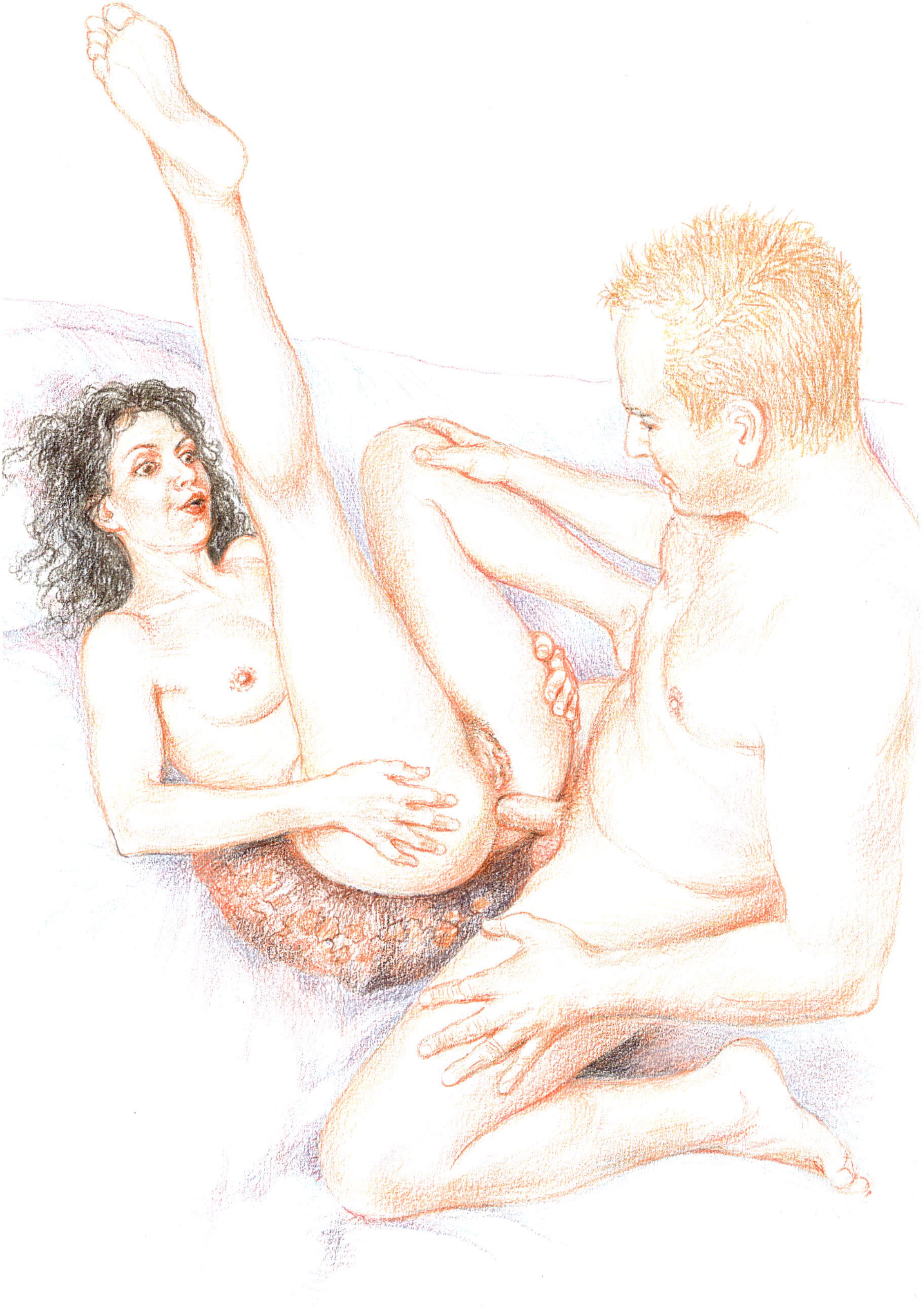

The Oyster

a dildo at the same time as having penetrative sex with a partner. A girl can have a lot of fun all on her own by using two dildos. Of course, two partners is the organic option and, if both of you are happy with this and you know someone you can ask, threesomes – and especially the two male, one female variety – are a great example of the whole being greater than the sum of its parts. There will be more on double penetration in our chapter on threesomes.

PIERCING AND TATTOOING

Piercing has already been dealt with earlier but deserves a mention here, as excessive piercing can be dangerous. And think about going through the metal detecting machine next time you fly off to some exotic place – you might have to show Airport Security more than you bargained for. Tattooing? Well, much of the effect can be achieved with transfers, so why should anyone need to have this eternal reminder that Tarquin or Elsie was once their flavour of the month? I mean no disrespect to the seriously pierced or tattooed, for they often make an art form of it, but the amateur should not undertake *either* of these forms of body adornment lightly.

WHEN BONDAGE BECOMES DANGEROUS

It may be that, as you explore and enjoy bondage as part of your sex play, you develop a taste for it and want to take it further.

As we mentioned before, with all bondage play it is the job of the 'top' to ensure that the 'bottom's' circulation is ok, that breathing is possible and that no choking is occurring. This is especially important where the 'bottom' might be spending a long time bound and gagged. And where the 'bottom' is in a particularly unnatural position, say, upside down, remember that the human circulatory system is miraculous but it takes a surprisingly short amount of time to disrupt it.

Be in no hurry, and discuss carefully with each other what you want out of the bondage: whether you want light restraint, something more stringent or total immobility. Talk about whether the 'bottom' wants to be hooded or blindfolded. And discuss the question of gags with great care. Some 'bottoms' find they like to be able to communicate verbally, some don't. Gags can be anything from a scarf that will restrict but not preclude speech, through tape across the mouth and rubber or leather bit gags to ball gags that have a rubber or metal ball fitting right inside the mouth. None of these would I personally recommend, but if you choose to use them, try them first and see how they affect your breathing before silencing yourself.

Once you are silenced, you lose your safe word, so you *must* have agreed some other form of sign that you wish the play to end.

EXTREME BONDAGE

At the expert end of the bondage scale are activities such as Japanese Rope Bondage – beautiful to look at, highly fetishistic and very complicated. The combinations and patterns of knots and bindings can take a long time to do and an almost equally long time to undo. So even to think about it, you have to be in a partnership where the sub is happy about spending a lot of time bound. There are many good, specialist books on Japanese Rope Bondage. Whether you wish merely to look and marvel, or to learn, do read them and work up from the simplest bindings to the more complicated if this appeals to you.

Also at the far end of the bondage spectrum are the people who like to indulge in almost complete sensory deprivation, a practice that can involve body bags and suspension. Again, there are specialist books on the subject, for these are highly specialised areas.

FISTING

This is the practice of introducing an entire hand and sometimes forearm into either the vagina. It should be approached with great care and is not generally regarded as a safe sexual practice. If you are consumed with curiosity by the possibility of fisting, there are specialist books on the subject and it would be a very good idea to get hold of one.

For our purposes here I will point out that, should you wish to go ahead and try it, there are some important precautions to be taken: the 'fister' should carefully check his or her fingernails for rough bits and hangnails and remove any jewellery. He or she may want to wear latex surgical gloves. And then… lubricate well and gently, very gently does it. The fister starts off with their hand flat and fingers pointed together, thumb

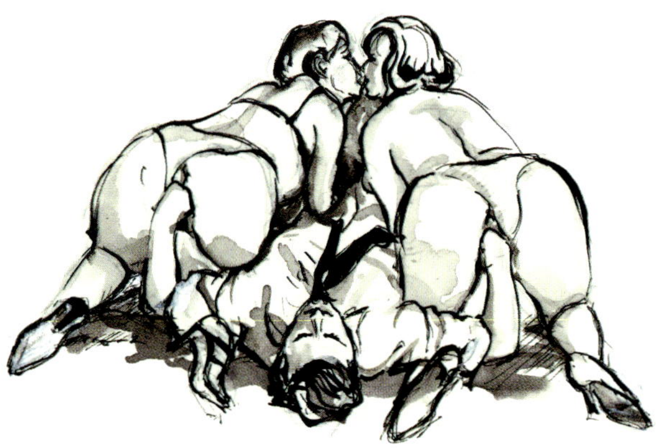

Double Fisting

tucked inside, entering the vagina with the palm facing their partner's stomach, but never her back – knuckles rubbing on the pubic bone feel most unpleasant. At this point, he should remind her to breathe deeply and relax. For those of you who wish to try anal fisting, the same sort of care must be taken.

If you do get to the stage of inserting the rest of your hand, let the knuckles follow and then overtake the fingertips until the hand inside forms a loose fist. Then, depending on what the 'fistee' wants and likes the 'fister' can clench and unclench his or her fist, spread the fingers and retract them again or gently 'punch' a little forwards and backwards. But be careful. Forceful pumping, or too fast a penetration and withdrawal can cause injury in various ways from air embolisms to removal of sections of the lower intestine. And the rectal wall is thin and delicate. It tears easily. The A&E Department of your local hospital is never a good place for a post-coital cigarette.

Fisting is an activity that must be based on great mutual trust and undertaken with great care and common sense. Be aware that some women may not be able to accomodate the whole hand, and older women, with thinner vaginal walls may find fisting painful. It is a hugely intimate thing to do, so I can't emphasise enough: be very sure and very careful before you even think of embarking on this.

DILDOS

Records of dildos go right back to ancient Greece and Egypt. French troops used to give them to their wives as a present before they marched off to war. From medieval nuns reportedly masturbating with altar candles and crucifixes, through Mick Jagger allegedly getting creative with serving suggestions for Mars Bars, down to Bill Clinton's way of ensuring

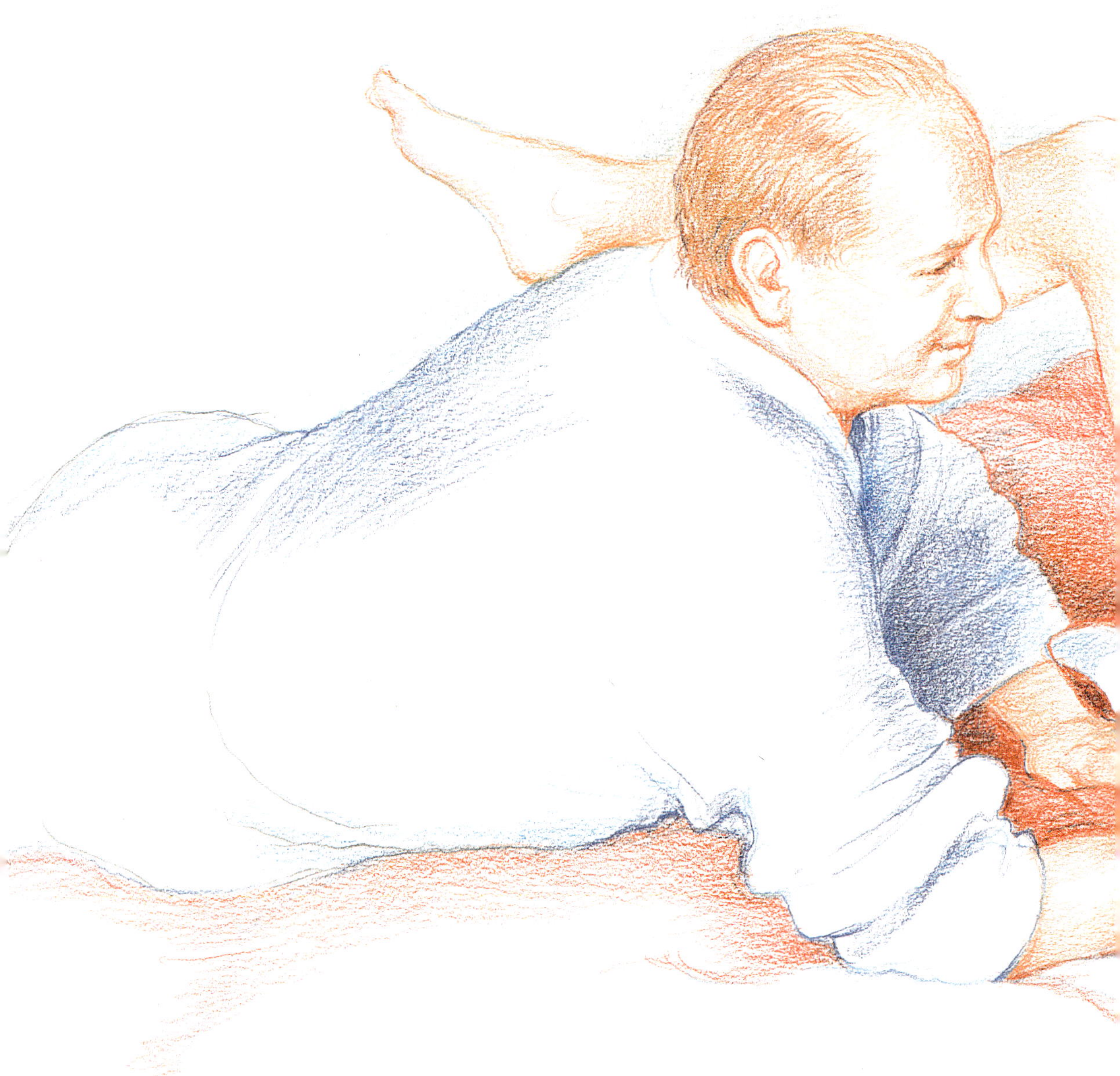

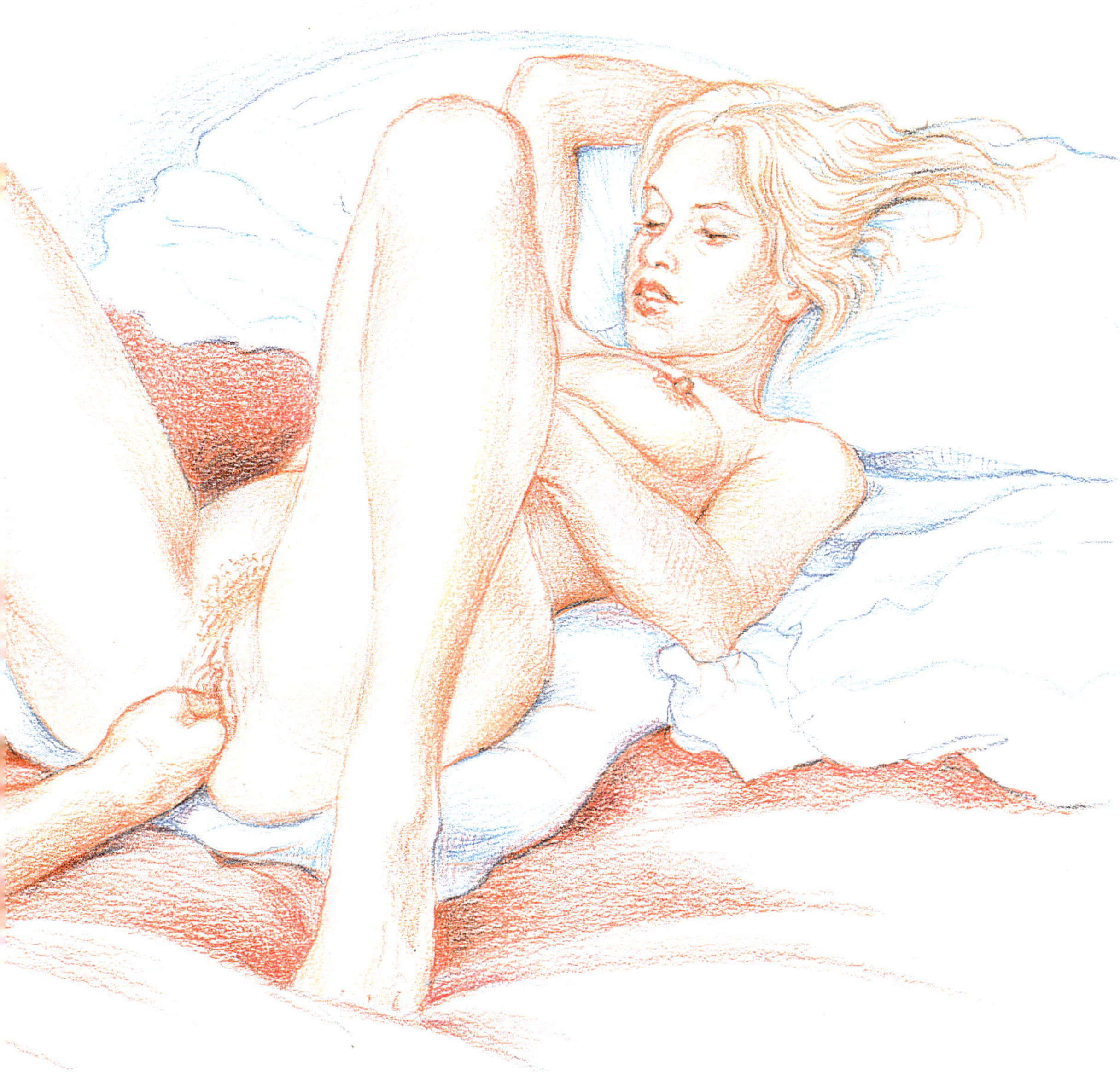

The fister starts off with
their hand flat and fingers
pointed together

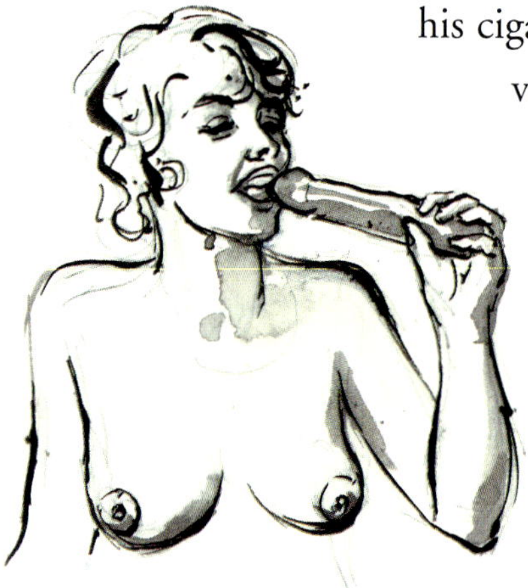

his cigars were nice and moist, people have sought variety and spontaneity in their sex toys. You only have to stand in a sex shop and look at the sizes, shapes, textures, materials and the colours on offer to appreciate that there's more to a dildo than you might think. There are even dildos cast from well-known willies so you can take the important parts of porn stars such as Jeff Stryker and Rocco Siffredi to bed with you.

And then there's the butt plugs, the anal beads, the double-headers and the rest. At the end of the day you will probably use what feels good for you – but you can have a lot of fun finding the perfect gadget. Insofar as shape and size is concerned, only you will know what hits the spot, and in terms of material, well, the world is your toy box. You can have anything from wonderful dildos available in Perspex, glass, and stainless steel to a well-scrubbed carrot or firm cucumber. Talking of which, the temperature thing that makes glass and steel dildos so sexy can be experienced by chilling a good firm cucumber, although it is probably a good idea to start with a courgette.

Historically, stone, clay, wax, ivory, rubber, fruit, vegetables, leather, and plastic have all been used. Dildos even get a mention in the bible:

Thou hast also taken thy fair jewels of my gold and of my silver, which I have given thee, and madest to thyself images of men, and didst commit whoredom with them. Ezekiel *16:17*

But there *are* a few basic rules where dildos are concerned: When you think about whatyou would like your plaything to be made of, be sure you are going to 'react' in the right way. Anything sugary, for example, will leave a residue in the vagina and can react with the bacteria there. Be aware that anything that leaves a residue can upset the biological balance of your vagina. Also anything that might flake or shed parts of itself can be a problem. Wood, or indeed glass, can leave nasty shards embedded, so check whatever you are using for cleanliness and integrity. Some people like a little roughness in texture, but I think we'd all agree that splinters are for those with specialist tastes.

CLEANLINESS IS GOODLINESS

If spontaneity is your thing, you must be sure that anything you or your partner grasp with erotic intent in the heat of the moment must be absolutely clean... which is not always the case.

THAT WHICH GOES IN MUST BE GETTABLE-OUTABLE

So anything that might break off, crush, melt or go mushy is a bad idea. It is not a great payoff to a little sexual adventure to spend time scooping the remains of your ripe banana or Cadbury's Flake from your undercarriage, despite what has been said about rock stars and their doxies. And, self-evidently, materials like glass should be avoided.

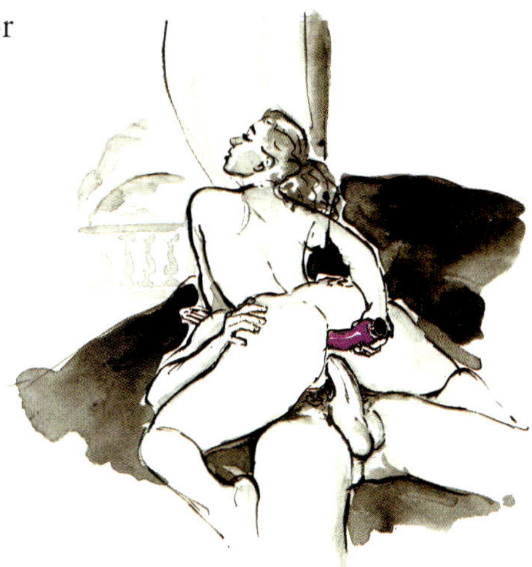

If you can't keep hold of it, have it on a

string: beads, balls and eggs in whatever material are great fun, but not if retrieving them is like finding soap in the bath. So a bunch of grapes (I'm not joking) isn't the greatest idea.

ELECTRICAL APPLIANCES

Of course, battery-operated vibrators are nothing new, but some people take it further and use household electric appliances. These are definitely a bad idea. Accidents have been reported involving everything from hand whisks and curling tongs to the hose attachment of a vacuum cleaner. At the risk of sounding like a killjoy, alive is better than dead, safe better than sorry.

ANAL TOYS

Look at a butt plug. It has a flange on the end of it, a flared section. Butt plugs and dildos are different and it is dangerous to use a simple dildo in your anus.

With its powerful rings of muscles, the anus, unlike the vagina, will simply swallow objects inserted into it – *almost* irretrievably!

The A&E departments of most hospitals have chapter, verse and X-ray on an amazing assortment of 'disappeared' objects. I have seen pictures of everything from a dildo that had slipped in – only to be followed by the pair of tongs with which someone tried to retrieve it – to a plastic doll. So, apart from observing all the caveats above, where anal devices are concerned, you must make sure that the insertion can be controlled and reversed.

EXPERIMENTS WITH GENDER REVERSAL

I have included this subject in this chapter for the simple reason that it can stir up extremely deep and disturbing feelings. To most of us our gender is set down at birth and remains an important part of our identity throughout our lives. However, there are occasions when the impulse to dress up as the opposite sex, just to see what kind of man or woman we would become, can be quite tempting. Mind you, it doesn't always have a good result; I knew one man who put on some female clothing and gazed in the mirror, hoping to see a delectable female replica of himself and instead saw a disturbing parody of his own mother, a lady with whom he had had a troubled relationship. The revelation shocked him and he never tried that experiment again.

Most of us swing between the two gender polarities in our emotions and we might feel limited by our physical bodies sometimes. Being a woman means being treated in a certain way, and having a female body means only being able to express feminine aspects, but how many of us have fantasised about bcing the one who overpowers and thrusts with masculine drive? I know I have explored these possibilities in my fantasies, but it is a more difficult matter to let them out in a real relationship.

I believe we need to be extremely secure in our own sexuality before we can begin to extend the boundaries. We all have preconceived notions of what is normal behaviour for men and women, but when you have been with a partner for sometime and become close to them it seems natural to want to try to know them at a greater depth and this can mean allowing them to let out the opposite side of their sexuality. I suppose we think first of all of a man wishing to dress up as a woman because there are so many fun garments for a man to delight in, not to mention wigs and make-up. It's much easier to add femininity to a man than make a woman look masculine, but psychologically it may be more of a risk for a man to take the plunge into a female guise. While he might add to himself in physical embellishments, he has to be prepared to give up some of his initiative by becoming sexually submissive.

Here is a completely honest account of how one man and his wife ventured into this ambiguous territory – and what happened as a result:

Marriage can be boring if you make it so: clean the car, mow the lawn, Eastenders *as a highlight. Trips to the supermarket, joining the pavement cattle grazing with their trolleys, have sex once a week... even missionaries had more imagination! Ten or twenty years into marriage, love can lose its passion and become overshadowed by domesticity. Unless, that is – you take a walk on the wild side.*

My wife has a best friend called Chloë. Chloë is all lipstick and lace. She likes other women, and that fascinates me. As I cleaned the car on Saturdays I had fantasies about Chloë, the car was always hers; same when I mowed the lawn on Sunday. The supermarket only became interesting when I pretended I pulled her *trolley.*

My wife of twenty years is capable of switching on a beguiling dominance that ends with obedience or dismissal. Some women are good at that, and secretly I found it attractive. A lot of men do. It's a power few women realise or use to their advantage.

On Chloë's suggestion, my wife once bought me a ladies' watch. I kept it on the desk, too dull to realise the subtle implications. (My brain had atrophied – all that missionary sex.)

I sat with my wife in a London pub, not much said. Two women close by made to leave. One kissed the other, not a peck on the cheek, but a brief, lipstick to lipstick, full-blooded bonding. I felt aroused and looked to my wife for comment, but went silent when I saw her eyes, rapturous concupiscence. An unguarded expression often shows a truth never spoken. I felt betrayed, then inadequate; I saw Chloë breast to breast with my wife.

Now I understood the implications of the ladies' watch, saw Chloë as counsellor, not rival.

In everybody's existence comes the opportunity to change, and if you remember the thrill of adolescent love, the passionate turmoil of mature love, the lingering fantasies lurking beneath the conventionalities of marriage, then you might try putting this sparkle into your life.

It's said that many men do it once, and most of these more than once. I had several times, in closet solitude, put on women's clothes. I love my wife, and have done since we first met. She was seventeen, I was twenty-two. She loves me (or so she says). Love is meant to live, a fiery passion between two souls, which encompasses, unconditionally, mind, body, spirit – and lust. When the opportunity comes to stir love, stir like crazy, because it doesn't happen often.

I'm slim in build and so is my wife, which helps. She was in the kitchen cooking dinner, and I knew she would be there for thirty minutes. I took the opportunity to dress with care, picked her favourite underwear, black lace knickers, suspender belt and bra. The bra was tight but the result was amazing. I had never realised that I was 'breasted'. The black stockings felt luxurious and the magical fastening of suspender tabs were the beginning of the metamorphosis. I chose an ankle length, black fitted skirt with elasticated waist. It clung like a web of sensuality. The grey silk blouse fitted fine, providing I left the cuffs loose and let the bodice reveal a trim little décolletage. I felt alive, on fire. The silver necklace and chain bracelet seemed enough, and I put my hair parting on the female side, backcombed and fluffed it a little, surprised at the result, as it gave me a softer face. I had no desire to look like a painted tart, so I applied a little lipstick and a generous spray of perfume. I was pleased with the result, I felt moist in my knickers. Now came the brave part. I shivered a little.

I heard of a wife who walked out on her husband after discovering him dressed in female clothes.My wife dropped the dinner. True, her mouth came open but only in the utterance of love. She had that same look of lust that I saw in the pub. My heart soared. In every man there is a woman and my femininity burst like a volcano. In her eyes, too, I saw myself as a woman. It changed our lives.

She took me to the living room laid me on cushions, kissed me gently, my cheeks, lips, neck and breasts, kissed me like she had never kissed before. Her power was absolute, my submission total. Her hand went under my skirt, over my stocking tops, lingered before she searched for what was tucked between my legs.

'As of now, it's a dildo,' she said. For an hour, these were the only words spoken. She eased it out, lifted her own skirt and settled herself down, pubic bone to pubic bone. I didn't think it was possible, but it was. She parted my legs so they came up, stockings clasped above her back. She began to pump on me. Oh bliss! This was heaven. Never again did I want to be a man. It had taken twenty years of marriage to discover our gender roles in one passionate outburst of love. Into my mind came a new world, a whole new relationship with all the thrill of discovery.

That was five years ago. I still clean the car and the grass still gets cut. Surprisingly, both of us cried that night, pent-up emotions released, joy, a feeling of pure adolescence, maybe. It felt good to be young again. Chloë calls occasionally, pats my bottom. I go down to the pub, drink beer, watch rugby. Male friends treat me no differently, how would they know? Women talk to me more, seem closer, tactile in friendly gestures. Underneath I bristle with female ambiguity. I shave my legs and body; trim my eyebrows, razor cut and bleach the hair on my arms. I exercise to develop my breasts. A small, subtle little handful, my wife says when she fondles me. Both of us exercise to keep trim. I take a size 12 skirt, 14 top. My wife loves to pamper me and I do the same for her. She buys all my lingerie; I've not worn male underwear since that night.

An old tree of love suddenly blossomed again, bearing new fruits. She has developed as the dominant partner and I'm content with female submissiveness; I've discovered it's my natural inclination. This realisation is like the lifting of a great weight. I wear female clothes in the house and garden. In public it's always male clothes on top, but sometimes slightly ambiguous – shirts and jeans, for instance. I have a relationship within in a marriage filled with love, communication and ambition. We talk about everything, from lipstick, to Byzantine art, to Wittgenstein.

My wife once had an affair with Chloë, but both broke away because of love and guilt. Chloë has four children. My wife bubbles in our relationship and regards me as a man and a woman in one, although she admits to an overwhelming preference for the woman. She taught me new ways to make love. I never knew my tongue was an instrument of rapturous bliss – plus the dildo gets good usage. Most of all she loves me role-playing as her maid. I tend her every need, all household and domestic chores. I have a couple of little maid's outfits: a tight micro skirt with white blouse and little frilly apron. Surprising what a maid and mistress can get up to.

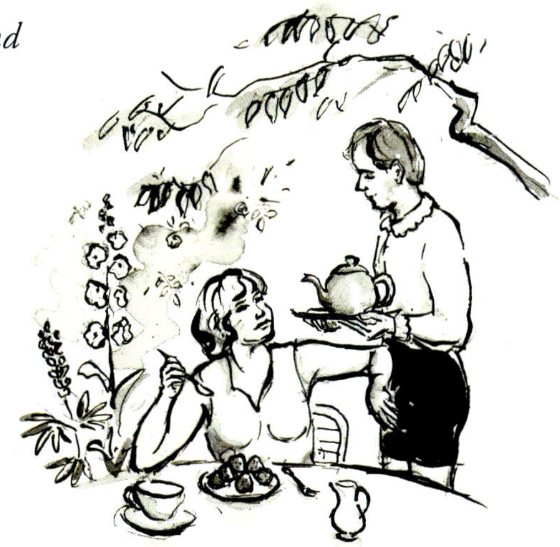

The writer of this account conveys well that moment when you are aware of the huge risk you take, but must still continue. As it happened, his decision was an inspired one; his wife entered in with an enthusiasm that even startled him. She could equally have taken one look at him and burst out laughing, making him feel thoroughly humiliated, never to try again.

Talking of laughter, I think it is wise to remember that there can be a lot of damage done by an inappropriate and untimely outburst. Joyous laughter, when it is shared, is fine, but sometimes we laugh simply because we are embarrassed or awkward, and this, more than anything else, can deflate and ruin any sort of erotic atmosphere. If a scene simply isn't working for you, it is always best to mention it tactfully at a later time when pulses have slowed down.

While the previous writer managed successfully to incarnate as his female counterpart, it seems that his wife remained in a female role, albeit more dominant, and they joined together in a special sort of lesbian coupling. This is probably the best way to experiment with reversals. It is nigh on impossible for a woman to be convincing playing the man when she is naked, even if she straps on a huge dildo and proceeds to fuck her partner.

STRAP-ONS

You can sample these unusual sensations without any dressing up or special role-play. If your man feels that he would like to experience a new, more empowered version of you, then why not go shopping together for a strap-on dildo. When you anally penetrate a man using a dildo, or just your finger, you will inevitably stimulate his prostate gland and many men find this a surprisingly pleasurable sensation.

i (This is the gland that contracts to release the seminal fluid before ejaculation. To find out more see *Sex Play* by Dr David Delvin.)

There are two different types of strap-on available: the harness variety which straps round the groin with some kind of O-ring where different sized dildoes may be fitted, and the all-in-one, where the 'penis' is permanently fixed to a harness or tightly fitting leather, rubber or PVC pants. For the beginner it is probably a good idea to use the adjustable variety so that you can start with a small dildo and work up to the size that suits you. The only drawback to these is that they do not always fit very snugly and this limits the amount of control you have over your newly acquired phallus. A man's genitals are superbly positioned on his body for the job they have to perform and we girls can often find that an artificial replica is never quite at the right angle; however, if you shop around you might find just the right one for you.

When you are choosing a strap-on, be aware that some materials are better than others. Avoid cheap plastic ones that are very inflexible. Rubber, though popular, flexible and attractively priced, is porous, which means it stains easily. Though more expensive than rubber, silicone is the best material; it is flexible, firm, smooth, strong and easy to clean. There is something sexy about its feel, making it nearer to the real thing than any other substance.

While you are getting your strap-on, don't forget to invest in a good quality lubricant too, see the section on anal sex for a list of good lubricants (p.128).

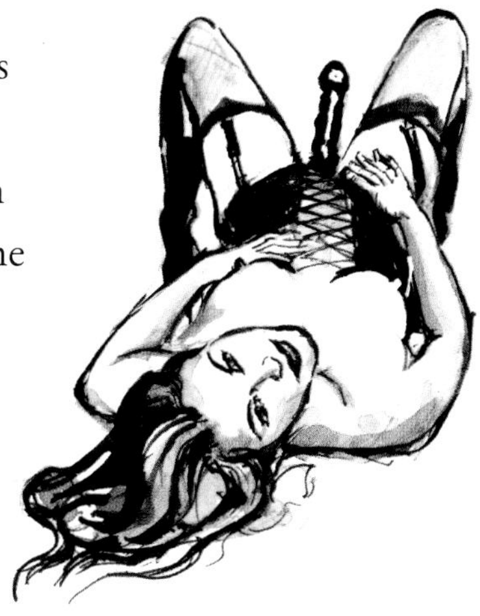

As I've already mentioned, for many men the anus and rectum are already erogenous areas, but just because this is so you must not assume that you can just strap on the strap-on and go to work. Unlike the vagina, the rectum does not have much natural lubrication so you must use plenty of 'lube'. The sphincter is a very powerful muscle (it needs to be for the job it does) and if it is not relaxed it must never be forced open. Force in this area can be excruciatingly painful.

Experimenting with a small butt plug for a few days first will help to prepare your man for what is to come.

Some men can be very apprehensive about having their arses fucked, imagining that it either won't stretch enough, or will remain open, leaving them incontinent. Neither of these fears have any foundation. Another understandable inhibition is due to the fact that we are dealing here with a potentially messy part of the body and inner cleanliness is vital. We also need to be aware of health issues (see section on anal sex, p.128).

There is another, very important reason for reservations. Such is the effect of centuries of socio-religio-sexual conditioning that many men's concept of hetero-masculinity is threatened by the idea of penetration. They never find out how much pleasure they can get because 'real men' don't have their bottoms played with, much less allow themselves to be fucked. Buggery and bottom-banditry smack of public school and jailhouse, submission and humiliation. 'Real Men' fuck and are not fucked. 'Real Men' are always Peg A, never Slot B. I have always felt sorry for these 'Real Men'. So be aware that for a man to accept your penetrating him – in any way – is an act of immense trust and intimacy. It is always best to go slowly.

To submit to penetration by another, even if it is a woman, may be associated for some men with homosexuality, especially if they are not very confident of their own virility. If this is the case, extreme sensitivity is needed.

When you put on your strap-on, leave it a bit loose to begin with as you will need to adjust its positioning to get the angle right for penetration. You can then tighten it up once you are inside. Prepare your lover by making him comfortable on his front and then start to stroke him between his buttocks. Using plenty of lubricant, gently slide a finger into his anus. It will probably open and then contract tightly around your finger. Wait until you feel the muscles relax, before inserting another finger and try to get the whole canal well lubricated, relaxed and open. Now put lots of lube onto your 'cock' and start to ease it slowly in. Don't force it in; you will find that the anal canal tilts forward slightly towards the navel and then turns back again towards the tailbone.

If your partner has never done this before he could be finding this experience a bit overwhelming and try to fight it. This will mean tensing up and immediate discomfort. To fully appreciate what you're doing to him, he must accept it completely and allow himself to open up. Take it easy at first; an initial bad experience can ruin any chance of further exploration.

Once your 'cock' has managed to gain entry you can start to gradually build up to harder and faster thrusts, but let the recipient guide you in this, because at first you won't have a clue. After a little practice, however, you will become aware of the amount of exhausting work that men put in when they are fucking you. And don't forget, it will be marvellous for toning up stomach and leg muscles. There is also a plus for females taking this dominant role – you can easily reach round and squeeze and play with his cock while you are penetrating him.

One tricky aspect to this is finding the right position. You'll have to experiment a bit. The most intimate position, and the one which will make the woman most aware of the role-reversal, is probably the one where your partner lies on his back and lifts his legs while you are on top, but he must be very fit to attempt that! All the other positions involve you both facing in the same direction, which means that you cannot gaze into each other's eyes – well, you can't always have everything. First of all, try it with him on his knees, doggy style, with you kneeling behind or lying over his back to fuck him. If this is too awkward a more comfortable position is the spooning one: both partners lie on their sides facing the same direction. This gives excellent access to your partner's genitals, or, you could both stand and simply bend him over the bed (see illustration).

Using a strap-on may not be to everyone's erotic taste, but it may provide an occasional excitement and if it enables you both to express a different side to yourselves then it will bring a new dimension to your sex life.

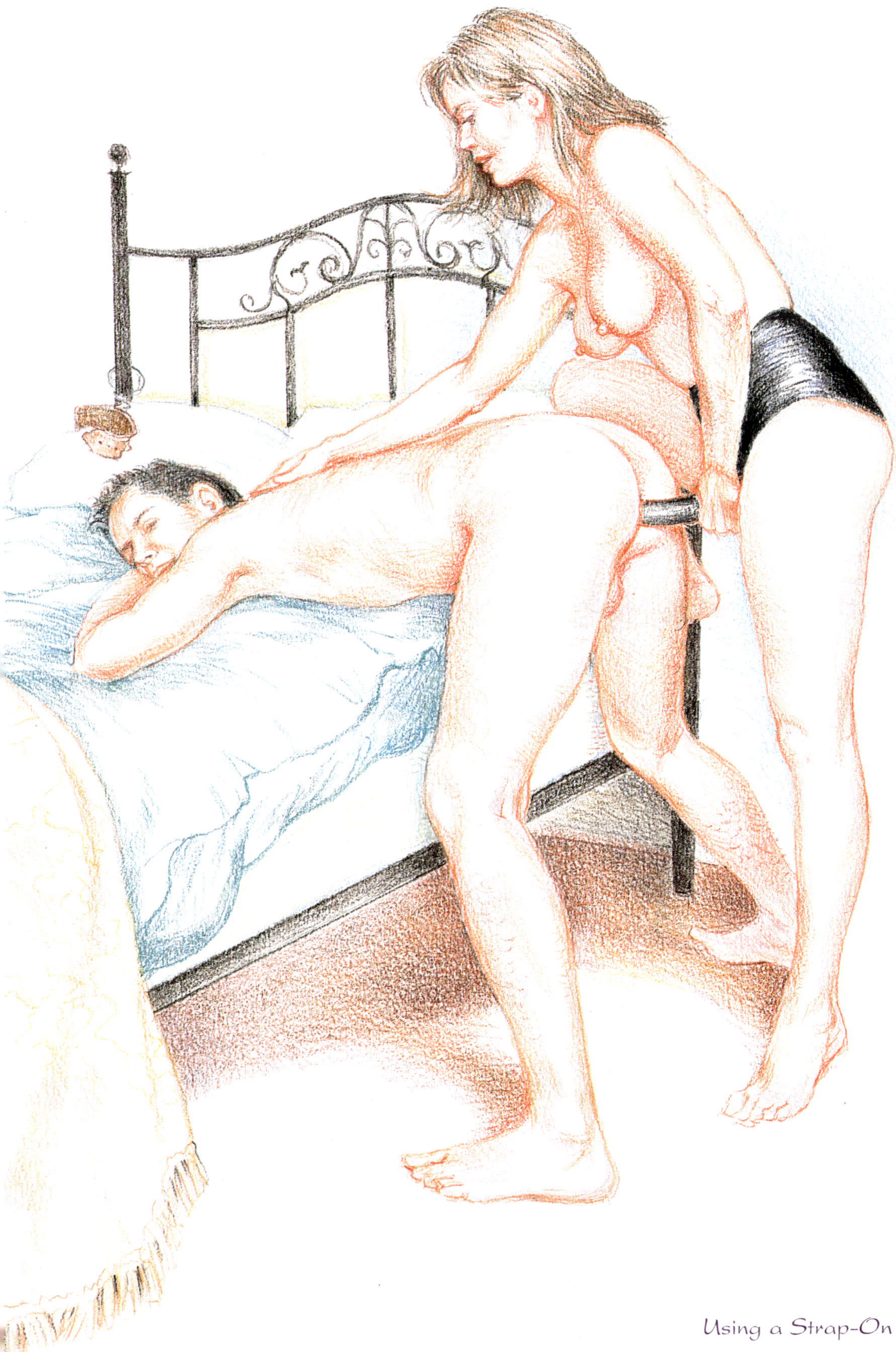

Using a Strap-On

5

including a friend

Nudism
Taking the Plunge
Contacts and Meeting People
Bisexuality and Threesomes
Finding a Like-Minded Couple
Swinging Parties
Clubs
Do Men and Women Have
Different Attitudes and Needs?

NUDISM

One way to gently break down barriers and inhibitions, if you happen to be a shy and physically modest person, is to try stripping off on a nudist beach, or at a sauna club, if they have naked evenings. Don't make the mistake, however, of assuming that a nudist club is a doorway to the more racy and sensual pursuits. You will be mightily disappointed, and probably deeply offend a few innocent nudists along the way.

Being able to be natural and relaxed while you are naked is an important advantage if you want to extend your sexual range and build your own confidence. To get you started, here are a few helpful tips from a committed nudist:

As a couple, you will undoubtedly have seen each other in the buff! In the raw! NAKED!! Under what circumstances? Making love, of course. Dressing and undressing in the bedroom. After all we don't live in the Victorian age, do we?

And yet there can still be a certain reserve. A feeling that nudity should be kept in its proper place and time. Like sex. For one or two nights a week perhaps, and certainly as part of the stimulus of sex. Maybe we feel that if we see too much of each other, it might lessen the sex drive, or perhaps we feel that our bodies, if revealed in full daylight might no longer be pleasing to our partner.

If we start living in the nude whenever possible, we learn to accept one another's body as part of that person, unique to him or her. There it all is, on show, and when the so-called ravages of time begin to take their toll, there is nothing to hide.

In what circumstances can we be naked together? Well, any and all, really. Watching telly; washing up; paying the electricity bill... (well, perhaps not in person, the world might not be quite ready for that yet).

Now, this is purely our view, but my partner and I feel that being naked together so much of the time has been a positive influence on our relationship. It's quite difficult to quarrel very seriously when neither of us is wearing the badge of authority, or the trousers, in the relationship or, in fact – anything at all.

The next step might be outdoors, in the sunshine, if any, or even in the rain. Have you ever stood completely nude in a deluge of rain? As a sensual experience it takes a lot of beating. As does swimming naked.

Now at this point I'm sure many people would say: what's the difference if I wear some covering in the storm, or a flimsy bit of material or two when I go swimming? For me, all the difference in the world. As a convinced nudist I simply could not bring myself to swim with anything on. I'd rather not swim at all.

So, where to now, then? Well, if your thing is streaking down the High Street, then anywhere at all. Otherwise, there are nudist beaches in many resorts, the most famous – but probably least pleasant – being Brighton. However, the Internet should provide you with a list.

You'll notice that I much prefer the word 'nudist' to 'naturist'. I find it self-explanatory and a lot less coy. However, now we're going to need that word because a great number of sun worshippers find that naturist clubs are ideal for them. I have to admit that they do have a lot going for them, especially if you have children. They usually have a swimming pool, a clubhouse and a cafe, and provide a very safe environment. By the way, young children are usually born nudists. When they become teenagers, well, that can be a different thing. Personally, I find that they can be rather falsely prudish. Many claim that there is no sexuality in naturism. I always thought there was sexuality in just about everything.

Phone British Naturism, or again – try the Internet for details. i

Oh, by the way, one for the guys. Will I get an erection the first time I see a naked female walking in my direction? The answer to this is that it's most unlikely, since you will be too nervous to think about anything. If you do have a worry about that, you could always position yourself strategically by the pool.

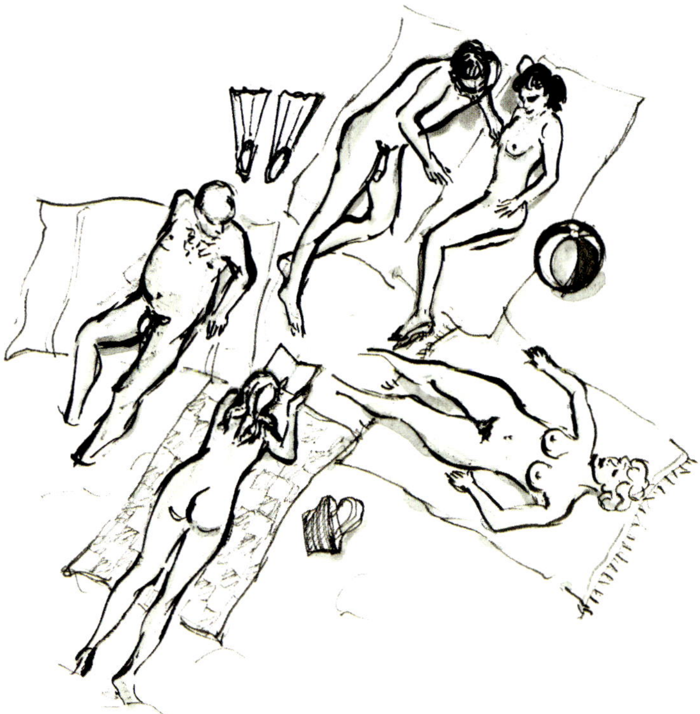

TAKING THE PLUNGE

Now we come to the section where there may be a dividing of the ways. I have been pondering this with trepidation. I thought that the best thing to do would be to give you the information, both the negative and the positive, and let you make up your own minds as to whether you wish to make the leap and say yes to involving real, live, other people in your sexual repertoire or keep it to just the two of you. It certainly *is* a big leap and can change your life forever, either adding spice and ecstasy beyond your wildest dreams or conversely, stirring you both up into a maelstrom of insecurities and resentment. To find out how you will react to seeing your partner sexually coiled with another, you need first to have got to the stage of complete honesty and sharing of fantasies. You need to be completely relaxed with the idea that he or she can be turned on by someone other than yourself, and above all there must be more to your relationship than just lust; you need to be very good friends indeed before you venture into these turbulent waters.

Swinging, as a philosophy, really got underway back in the late 60s with the hippy movement and probably had its joyous heyday in the 70s, before AIDS put in its unwelcome appearance. Back in those days there were idealistic explorers who were trying to understand and acknowledge the reality

Swinging Experiences: Deborah and Adam

Paula Did you find yourself in the swinging scene by chance, did it happen spontaneously, or did you make a concerted effort?

Debbie A concerted effort. We talked about our thoughts and fantasies.

P Did you fantasise about somebody else joining you?

D Yes, another girl joining. The classic threesome really.

P Did you find a girl?

D Well, we placed an advert in a contact magazine and found a couple.
Adam We soon discovered that there are very few single women...
D ...and having had the first experience, which I was very lucky with because they were an older couple, and she was very 'bi' – I hadn't thought of myself being very that way – it just went so well.

P You weren't bothered by this discovery? Would you say you are very secure in your own sexuality?

D I am the sort of person that once I've decided on something then I don't think of anything negative. So I dived in – and that was it.

P What did you think about the girls together?

A It's every man's fantasy, I suppose.

P Why do men love that so much?

A Well, two things really: one is that you see it from a different angle – but it's definitely not just a voyeuristic thing because I always want to be in the middle of it.

D True, if we are there sharing with him it's not as threatening as if we went off somewhere together.

A And I think it goes back to our school days when we used to wonder about sex and how to do it, and girls were always supposed to know more about it than we did so obviously if you can watch two girls together they are going to show me what they like.

P That's a very good point. Casting your mind back to the beginning, how long had you been together before you started swinging?

D Well, we had both experimented sexually before we met each other, but once our relationship had started we had to wait until it was strong enough. You have to know that your relationship is strong before you can bring somebody else in because if there is a weakness you can't expect that swinging is going to mend the relationship; it has to be something to enhance it.

A That is the big mistake people make. We've met couples who have had a serious problem with their relationship and think that swinging is going to fix it, and it never works.

P Can swinging help contain a couple's need for variety, provided they both remain focused on each other?

of human sexuality in its natural form, and break away from the artificiality and dishonesty of most marriages. Quite a tall order, for no one really knows what natural man or woman would be like if they stopped lacing themselves into sexual straitjackets. Would they be lolling around self-indulgently copulating all day long, like some kinds of near-human apes have been observed to do? Or would they be like many other mammals, with dominant males running harems of females and fighting off all other males who tried to break in? I don't know, but we've all noticed these traits in humans – the self-indulgence and the possessiveness. If you are going to find pleasure in a new sexual morality (there have to be some sort of rules laid down, as any committed swinger will tell you), both these traits must be mastered. But, try to retain the ape's natural spirit of co-operation and general lustiness.

When couples let down their barriers and enter into sexual encounters with others for the first time, the relief can be exhilarating for they find that they are not alone. They feel that they have been admitted into a sort of commune where honesty, sharing and generosity are taken for granted. They discover that in general, in the world outside, hardly anyone is ever completely honest about their sexuality.

CONTACTS AND MEETING PEOPLE

Sex is always so inextricably linked with power that you have to be careful how you go about finding new playmates and try not to exploit people or be exploited yourself. The safest way seems to be by contact advertisements where you can be clear about what you are looking for and everyone knows where they are.

Many years ago I used to be a paste-up artist for a contact magazine called *Experience*, now sadly killed off, and it always amazed me to see how uninhibited some people were prepared to be in the photographs they sent in – provided their faces had a small triangle cut out of them obliterating any recognisable facial features. The physical

A Only if that couple still enjoy being together, because we've met couples and it's been abundantly clear that one of them is just doing it to keep the other one happy, in case they might wander off and have an affair, or maybe their life may have become boring and tedious.

P So you're saying that you must never make a dull love life the reason for doing it?

It wasn't that you were bored with each other?

D No, certainly not! We already had an exciting love life but this enhanced it…

A The idea is that we do things and then fantasise that other people will join us. If you have a vivid imagination there's a limit to how much two people can do. The more people who get involved the more combinations there are!

D Also, you can have really good sex between the two of you but it's nice sometimes to have 'fun' sex with others, without the deep down emotion… because it IS different. If you're fond of games and role-playing it's quite nice to have someone else doing it with you. Some of the people we've met have gone on to become really good friends but there are those who are short burst encounters. They aren't really on the same wavelength; we might enjoy sex with them briefly but we wouldn't want to live our lives around them.

A People we have the least in common with are those who take it all too seriously. Some of them are so tense, and consuming…

D I think it's important not to continue something if it's not giving you pleasure. I believe strongly that both partners must be happy with what they are doing; if one of you isn't then it's no good.

A Yes, that's one of the rules we've always had.

D We met an extremely nice couple, and I got on well physically with the man, but Adam isn't particularly keen on lots of pubic hair. Well, this girl was really hairy...

A It was probably what turned her partner on...

D But unfortunately Adam found this a bit of a turn off. I was having a good evening but when I realised that he wasn't, that was the end of it... I rang the man afterwards and said I would be happy to meet them alone for a threesome, if they liked.

P Did you mind Debbie going off for a threesome without you?

A No, not at all. My only reservation though was that the woman was very bi and her partner was rather possessive. When we had tried to get involved as a foursome we were all on the double bed, two couples, one on each side, me with the other woman. We moved over a bit towards Debbie's side because I knew she would enjoy having contact with the woman – she is very 'bi' – but then he went to the floor by the bed and made Debbie move away from us; then as we moved to the edge of the bed we found both of them were on the floor. I tried to make it possible for the two girls to have contact but the next thing we knew he had taken Debbie out of the room onto the landing. We ended up practically chasing them around the house...

bodies were all shapes and sizes, which I found reassuring, for here were *ordinary* people – not models. I know that contact ads and the type of terms and language used can be the butt of many a joke. Some of the images can be quite raw and off-putting, but in spite of this humorous (some might say undignified) aspect, I still think that advertising is the best way to find the people you are looking for.

You may not respond favourably to all those who answer your advert but you can choose carefully who you both wish to meet, and need not tell anyone where you live until you are on a firm footing with them. Always meet new people in a public place first and see how you get on. Whatever happens, you will have your partner with you and can check out each other's reactions after a meeting. If anything develops, you will be able to look after each other and feel secure. You don't need to rush into intimacy. Take your time and get to know a little about any new contact by phone or email before you decide to meet again. Some of these new acquaintances could develop later into real friends, but it's more likely that they will be ships that pass in the night, for even if you have a similar sexual preference to someone else and find them physically attractive, this doesn't necessarily mean that you have anything else in common. But where friendships *do* spring up, they will be close and enduring.

Years ago, I must confess that I could not believe that swinging and orgies and other unconventional erotic group activities ever actually happened. It was often insinuated, with a nudge and a wink, that an orgy had happened last week or last night, but it always remained a mystery as to who had organised it and what had taken place. Tentative people sometimes tried to push situations as far as they could, but they always withdrew before anything really interesting happened. When you first find out that all these extraordinary things *do* occur, and on a much wider scale than you could have imagined, you start to wonder why you never met anybody before who was involved in

D That's another thing: if you know that your partner particularly likes something then obviously you'll steer things in that direction so that they get as much pleasure out of it as possible. It's a feature of partnership: not just doing it for your own pleasure. Obviously, it wasn't going to work with that couple.

A That was an example there... because of the physical lack of attraction I couldn't get an erection. This became an issue: with a foursome that sort of thing only becomes an issue if you separate into couples. It was then a case of 'you're well away and we're at the other end of the bed with nothing happening'. When Debbie joined us it became fun again. That's why it didn't work.

D While we're talking about relationships, you have to be quite strong to know what your partner wants and expects from swinging. It's no good entering this scene on a whim. You really need to discuss beforehand what each couple expects – whether they want to be together or in separate rooms – so that there are no awkward moments.

A What I personally like doing is meeting first as a four, then if it works, to split up and go into separate rooms and then come back together again. Because there are people, particularly first timers, who are a bit nervous and who are often doing it for the benefit of their partner. I find, if I take another woman aside, I can actually find out what she likes.

D But then, you are a very attentive lover...

A Yes, but I can only be an attentive lover if I know what they enjoy...

P On the other hand, if you're taking them off and helping them, their husband isn't seeing what you're doing, to learn from it too. You might be introducing an element of competition there...

A Yes, I suppose that is a danger.
D But, if you have a strong relationship, you can benefit by doing different things with other people.
A Yes... like anal sex for example. It's quite common in a loving relationship that one or other partner won't like doing it. Now here is a new lover, and maybe they would like to do it, because their own partner doesn't want to.

P True, I know someone who likes spanking very much but his wife doesn't enjoy it so she is quite happy for him to find someone who does. It's much better than her just grinning and bearing it, which wouldn't give him any pleasure at all.

D That's the main thing – if you can accept that your partner is enjoying it but they aren't mentally detached from you, the affection hasn't gone,
A We see it like... going out and having a meal with friends: the sex is just like the fifth course. It's NOT like falling in love or wanting to run away with them or anything like that. We enjoy socialising and chatting and so on, and this is just the next stage on. I know some find that difficult to understand.

P Yes they do. Many people feel that sex is just a private activity between two people and that involving others could cause disatisfaction.

such adventures and then you wonder whether you already have, and they just never mention it to you!

Place an ad in a magazine or through the Internet and you will be amazed at the response you will get. You could be inundated with new possibilities, but I would strongly suggest that you read the two interviews included in this section and take note of the advice given by these experienced couples, for they have both had their emotional ups and downs. If your relationship is not firmly based and strong enough to withstand outside influences, it could be stretched to breaking point.

Experienced swingers who have managed to stay happy and fulfilled will always say that it is *vital* to discuss all your reactions and concerns at every stage of the way so that you both know exactly where you are going. And it's also more crucial than ever that you take full responsibility for your health and do not take foolhardy risks by having unprotected sex with strangers you know next to nothing about.

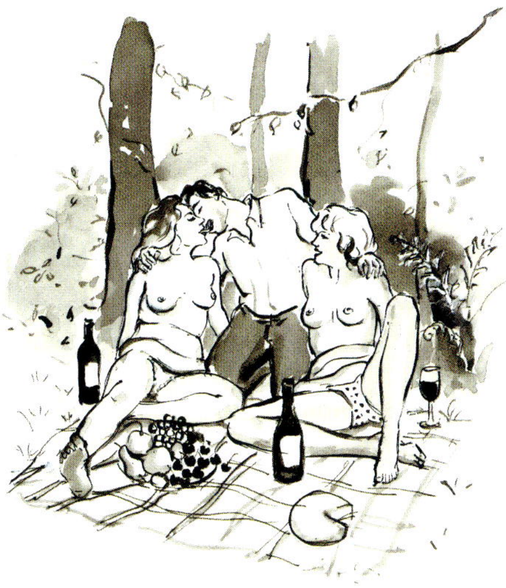

BISEXUALITY AND THREESOMES

One of the first issues to be dealt with when you start out will certainly be bisexuality. Up until now, if you are a newcomer, you probably will not ever have been close to a naked member of your own sex in an erotic atmosphere. You will soon find out how you react. Let's take the female point of view first. Here are the observations of one highly experienced woman:

It's the oldest male fantasy in the book; a candle lit bedroom, soft music playing,

D Yes, there can be resentment... Also, I have noticed with some people, that they can't get to grips with the messiness of sex. But it shouldn't matter. You end up in the shower or the bath, which can be equally enjoyable. The thing is, not to get hung up about how you look. Your make-up runs, you sweat a bit, and sometimes you wind up with cum in your hair. The main thing is that you enjoy yourself. Have fun, and if you make funny noises, just laugh!

A Don't be embarrassed.

D People have this idea that it has to be like in the storybooks; all wonderful, but actually, sex is quite raw really.

A One more thing: having the confidence in yourself so that it doesn't matter if somebody else is better than you at something... I mean I really don't mind.

P I think you are pretty unusual there.

D Having self-confidence is important... I find it difficult to express when people ask me how I do it – I can't really explain – I am just naturally very open. You just have to let go a bit.

A When one of us comes up with a new idea the response the other one gives is automatically 'yes!' It doesn't mean to say we are going to do it, but the immediate response is positive. We might decide – hang on, it's not very practical and maybe it doesn't happen, but Debbie will always say `Yes, OK, let's try.' There are some people whose immediate reaction will always be 'No'. They may think about it, but...

D Their partners will assume they

aren't keen and it will put them off.

A Whereas, if you can embrace a new idea... OK, it may not be practical – some of the things we have concocted are never going to happen, there is no way they could...

P Thinking about couples coming to all this for the first time, perhaps we should advise them to start off very gradually.

D Oh, definitely! First of all you need to learn to open up with each other – a lot of couples won't even share sex magazines together and I have friends who get annoyed if their husband looks at porn sites on the Internet. If you can sit in bed together, with some magazines... I used to do that with my first husband. We wouldn't read the stories out loud because that would spoil our private pleasure, but we would both get turned on by a story and then it would go from there; you get ideas for fantasies from the stories – some were quite explicit.

A But there are women who are quite unhappy with their physical appearance and the concept of their husband getting turned on by looking at someone else in a girly magazine makes them resentful.

P I think it's lovely when a man can look at a picture and say to his wife, 'Look, isn't she gorgeous!' and the wife to say, 'Yes she is!' – or just someone walking down the street, and the wife might say, 'What a lovely arse he has...'.

D Yes – exactly; I think it's a starting point. After that you might look at some toys and at the reader's wives sections in

him, you – and your best friend; or the girl from the office, or possibly Catherine Zeta Jones. The stuff of a thousand 'Letters to the Editor' in sex mags, and a hundred thousand porn videos!

All men love the idea of female bisexuality, however ambivalent they might feel about it with their own sex; but how does it feel to be a bi-lady, and what actually happens when three in a bed equals one man and two women? I suspect that it is answering these questions that puts more people off trying it out than actual distaste for the idea.

First, let me say that not all threesomes involve bisexuality, and there is no reason why two bisexual ladies can't have sex together without spectators; I can only speak from experience: most of the sex I have had with other ladies has involved an audience of at least one – and very frequently more.

The first time I made love to another woman was at the grand old age of 42. I had been a happy hetero all my life, but I felt that this was something I had to try, at least. If I didn't like it, so what? I hadn't liked skiing either, but giving it a shot hadn't left me traumatised for life. So the ad was answered ('husband to watch and join in if invited'), the date was made, and a lovely blonde vision in a black velvet miniskirt showed me how ladies do it to ladies.

I was surprised to find how easy it was; not all women want to go all the way the first time, but I found one thing led very naturally to another, and before I knew it, there I was – eyeball to eyeball with my first open pussy. The subject of how to give pleasure to a woman using one's hands and mouth has been so extensively covered elsewhere that I'm sure no-one needs my contribution, but the important thing was that it was delicious, that it was fun, and that making her come still ranks as one of my great personal achievements. All you have to do is to think about what you really like, and make it happen to her – the sense of empathy, of sharing something as intimate and complex as a female orgasm is a buzz that you don't quite get from any other sexual experience.

Other women feel nice, they smell nice, and they notice and compliment you on your new sexy underwear. They are also

magazines to see what others get up to, and finally start looking at the contact section. It develops from there really.

P Preparation is very important...

D And talking about your fantasies.

A Unfortunately a lot of women DO have hang-ups about the way they look – their boobs aren't big enough, or their bums are too big or whatever. Most women would want to change something about themselves but it shouldn't matter... If Debbie sees me looking at a photo of another woman who has a bigger chest than she has it won't bother her because she doesn't suffer from insecurity. The moment you go into swinging you are going to find others that are more attractive than you are – at a party there is always bound to be someone – and if you see your partner with a woman or man who is more physically perfect than you, if you are an insecure person, it could be disastrous.

P Let's get back to the subject of threesomes. Have you found it difficult to find the ideal person to bring in?

A We usually only meet up with couples; that's the way it has been. You remember the couple we talked about just now? Well, as I said, Debbie phoned up the man and said that since I wasn't very interested, would they like her to join them for a threesome? They turned her down flat!

P Oh, they didn't!

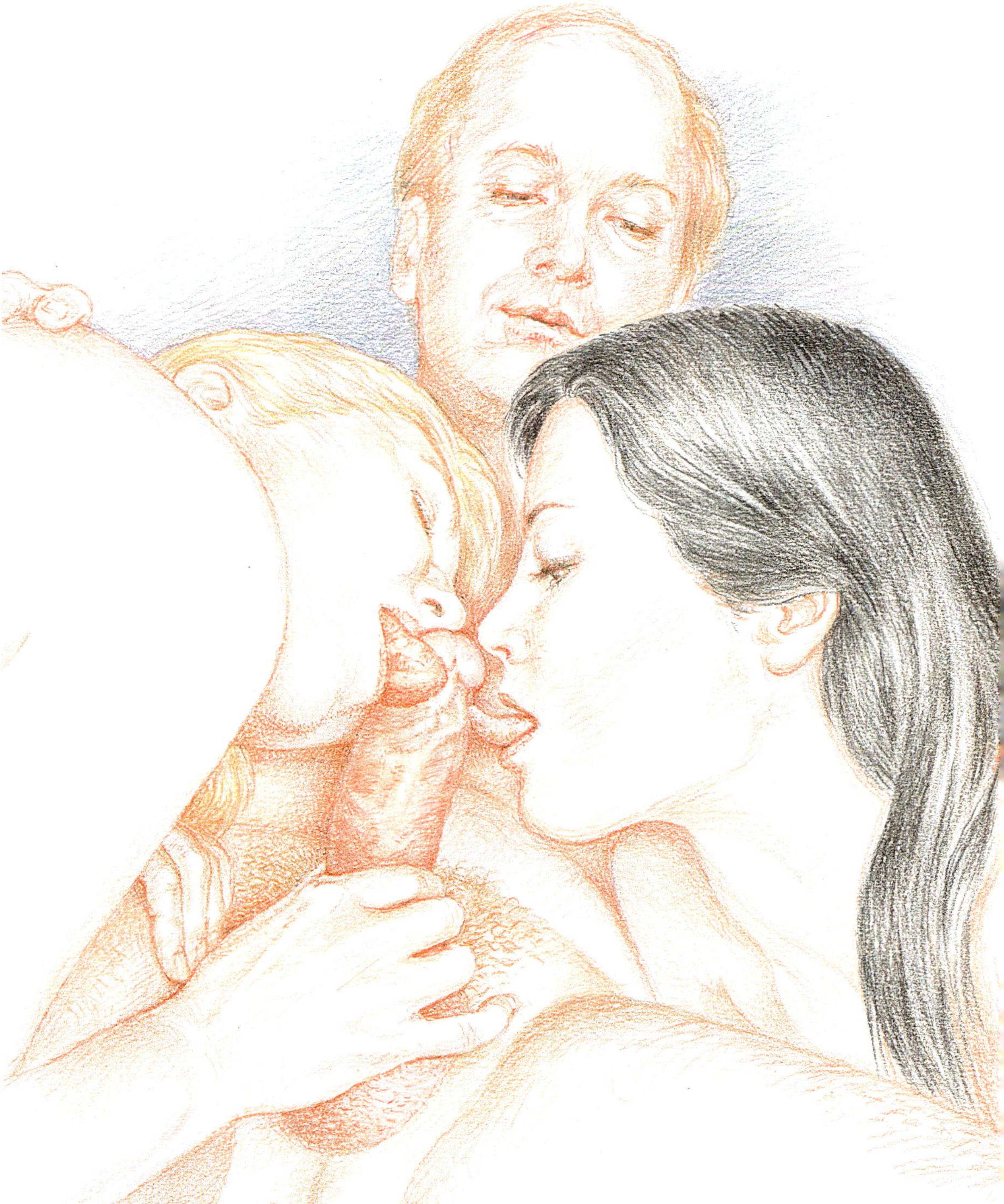

prepared to spend as long as you need on cunnilingus, because they aren't being distracted (as men can be) by the urgent demands of an erection! They aren't down there for any other reason than that they like it, and they like you.

Girl-on-girl sex can cover a very wide range of activities, from just kissing and stroking, to full-on oral, and penetrative sex using a vibrator or strap-on, right through to bondage, spanking and fantasy role playing as described elsewhere in this book. Some women may even find it easier to initially explore some of their wilder fantasies with another woman, as

D Yes, he said – and I don't know if he even consulted his partner – that they preferred to keep it to couples because that way they wouldn't endanger their relationship.

A I think he noticed that you two ladies were attracted to each other and if you had joined them he would have had to take a back seat. I don't think he could have taken that.

D We do have one girl who joins us occasionally and it works very well. We're old friends and we all know what each of us likes. Adam is such a considerate lover and there is equal sharing. Sometimes they both make a fuss of me and it's wonderful.

P How did you meet this lady?

A We met originally with her and her partner, then when the relationship split up we kept on with her. The split was nothing to do with us, by the way. We tried to keep friendly with them both, but eventually it became too complicated and we had to make a choice. The three of us have become very close.

D We've been lucky. I can remember a girl – this was before Adam – she was Norwegian and very open-minded. We had one of those double-ended dildoes – and some vibrating ones too. That was marvellous. But of course there are so many more things you can do when a third person is there.

P While two of you are fucking, the other can come up behind and use their tongue...

D Yes we've tried all that. Not just tongues, dildoes too.

P Do you use it on him, might I ask?

D Yes I do... but there are lots of guys who don't go for that. It's something that has gradually developed with us.

P I think a lot of men probably couldn't accept a role reversal.

A No...but that came more from Debbie than me...
D We used to just play around at first, and you thought, 'Mmm... that feels nice!' – and of course you had some erotic books and we'd seen pictures – so for me it wasn't such an alien thing to consider. I don't remember how it developed.
A I remember you using the strap-on on me for the first time, and it was actually you who suggested it...

P It must be quite hard to find one that straps on properly. I mean men are beautifully designed to be just at the right angle and penetrate in the right place! But with strap-ons you can find that they stick out at the wrong angle and shift around and bend.

D Oh no! We've got an absolutely wonderful one!
A It's a very expensive one – the cost was in three figures.
D It's leather and you never feel like you've got it on. Once you're wearing it, it moulds itself to your body.
A It's all properly shaped and sits on your hip.

P Do you like going to sex shops together? That's something couples don't often do together.

our first 'make believe' games when we were little girls were often with same-sex friends.

Having said that, lots of bi-ladies feel more comfortable when there's a man around (after all, they are so good at opening the champagne), and the gentleman (or even the men) in your life will almost certainly find watching you together a thrilling experience.

Now you guys, if you are lucky enough to have your sexy woman put on a show for you with her lovely friend, then bear in mind that there are rules. I'm serious here. You are in for a big treat, make no mistake, and you will ruin it – perhaps forever – if you charge in like an overheated bull in a china shop, and start sticking your bits where they aren't wanted: so Rule Number One is 'Front End Planning'. Talk it through first. Are you going to just look, are you going to be allowed to touch, and if so who, and when? Maybe your partner doesn't want you playing with her friend; maybe her friend doesn't fancy the idea (yes, I know you and your woman both think you are utterly *irresistible, but sadly different*

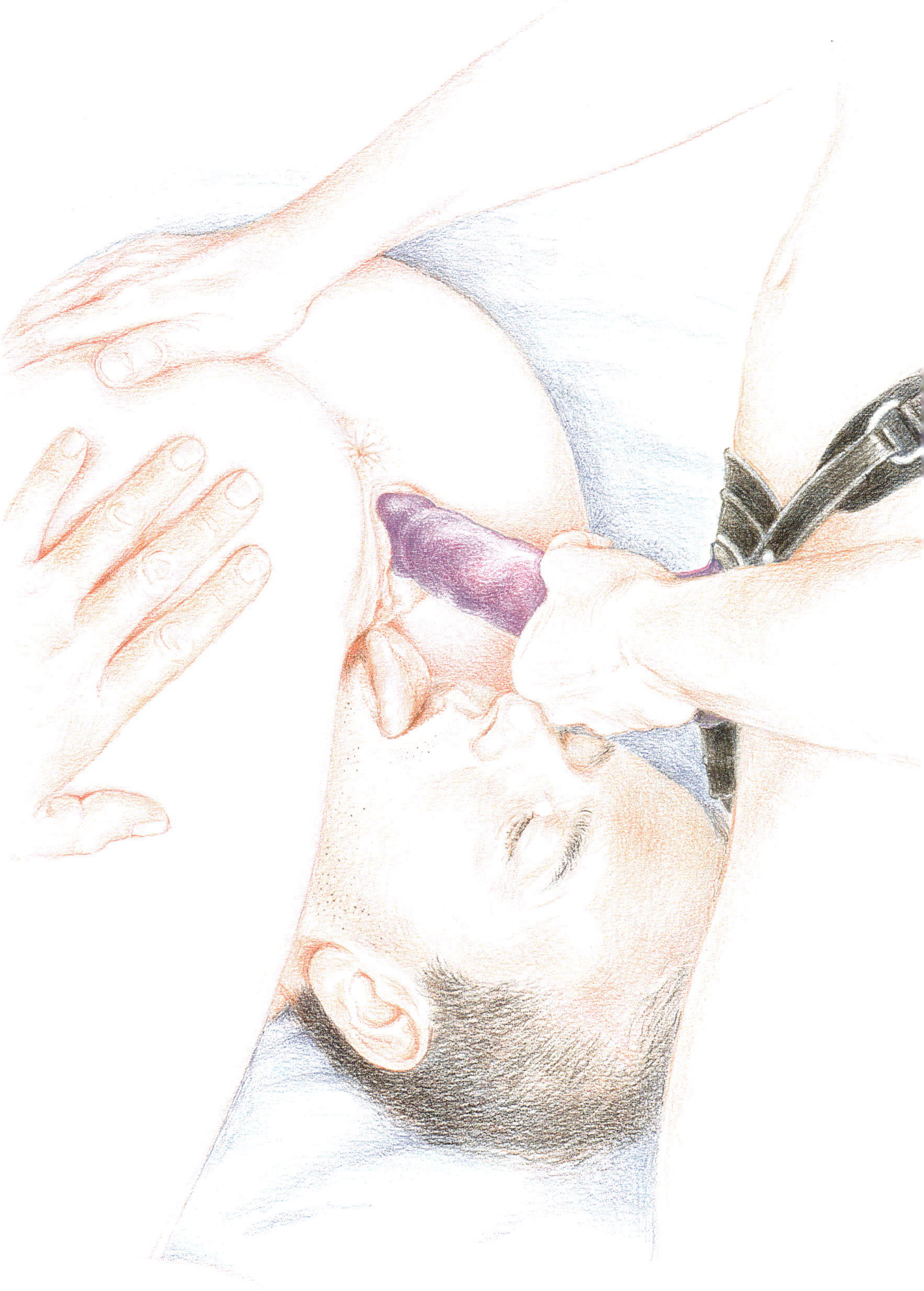

D No, we mainly look at things on the Internet together and use mail order. I think it's good if people can buy playthings together because it all adds so much to the pleasure they can have.

P What sort of scenarios do you like?

A There was the picnic bench...
D Oh yes! Last year we did get completely carried away. Adam had rung me at the last minute and said meet me at the picnic bench.
A This place is in the middle of the woods; it's a big picnic site...
D At night it's completely dark. There is literally no lighting – except for moonlight.
A It's completely in the middle of nowhere.
D This particular night we were both extremely turned on. The moon was shining and it was very warm. I ended up completely naked. You were too and I bent you over the bench and ended up doing you from behind, wearing our special strap-on! We were really making a lot of noise.

P I take it that no one was around?

D No, well, to be perfectly honest, I wouldn't have noticed! It always turns us on to think that someone might...

P That adventure sounds lovely. Especially as it was such a balmy night...

D Yes... we've done lots of things but that was one of our special times. We laughed so much too. We were really intense while we were

people have different tastes). None of this has to be a problem if you all talk it over lovingly and frankly before *anything happens.*

Having set the ground rules, Rule Number Two is 'Patience'. You are going to be in close proximity to two gorgeous bodies, four bouncing boobs and luscious thighs, two peachy bottoms and succulent pussies. This is not a film – it's real life. You may be filled with the urge to make gorilla noises and throw yourself into the fray; resist it. Wait until you are invited, however long it may take, and when you are invited, remember the territorial limits the three of you agreed earlier.

The Third Rule is 'Awareness'. Even if you are sticking to the ground rules, if either lady looks the slightest bit uncomfortable, back off. People aren't always aware of their own limitations; the sight of you going down on another woman might make your partner feel hurt and jealous, even if she previously thought it would be fun, or the other girl might find at the last minute that she isn't happy about being penetrated by you. Be alert, be empathetic, and be ready to change tack and give either or both ladies a big hug and reach for your boxers with good humour and a good grace if it all goes wrong!

The Fourth and final Rule is 'Appreciation'. You think they look fabulous? Tell them! You're having the time of your life? Say so! Every woman wants to be a sex goddess sometimes, and here is your opportunity to convince two at the same time that they are the stuff of erotic dreams: unless you don't feel like that of course, in which case you will probably find that old Hornby train set is still in the attic somewhere...

Now then girls, what do we do with this big steamy chunk of testosterone that has joined us on the bed, eyes slightly bulging and breathing heavily? Well, presumably we wanted him there in the first place, so he's entitled to have a bit of a fuss made of him. Depending on what you agreed before, one or both ladies can start kissing and stroking him; his partner may describe his most erogenous zones to her friend, and show her how to stimulate him. Try going down on him together (great fun if someone remembered the

doing it, anyone could have come up, but afterwards I climbed up on the table and laughed, both of us completely starkers.

A It was wonderful.

D It's nice that we can change round, not have one of us dominating all the time.

P You aren't a particularly dominant person are you, Adam?

A No, not really...

D If anything, you tend to be very content to give me pleasure.

A Yes... I could play the role of being masterful, but it would be something I'd have to work at.

P And of course that wouldn't be what you wanted, Debbie.

D No, I don't think I am naturally domineering, but if someone responds to me that way, I can completely throw myself into it. If I say to someone 'come here, naughty boy', and they respond in the appropriate way then I can get into it, but if there is no response, then I just drop it.

A It has to be spontaneous... like that evening in the wood; you knew exactly what you wanted to do. You got a great deal of pleasure out of it and so did I and we're so comfortable in our relationship, I didn't have to worry about thinking 'I've got to make sure she comes...'

D No; that evening was completely for you!

A That's what it comes back to; we want to give pleasure to each other.

P That's something that can't be taught. I'm sure many people

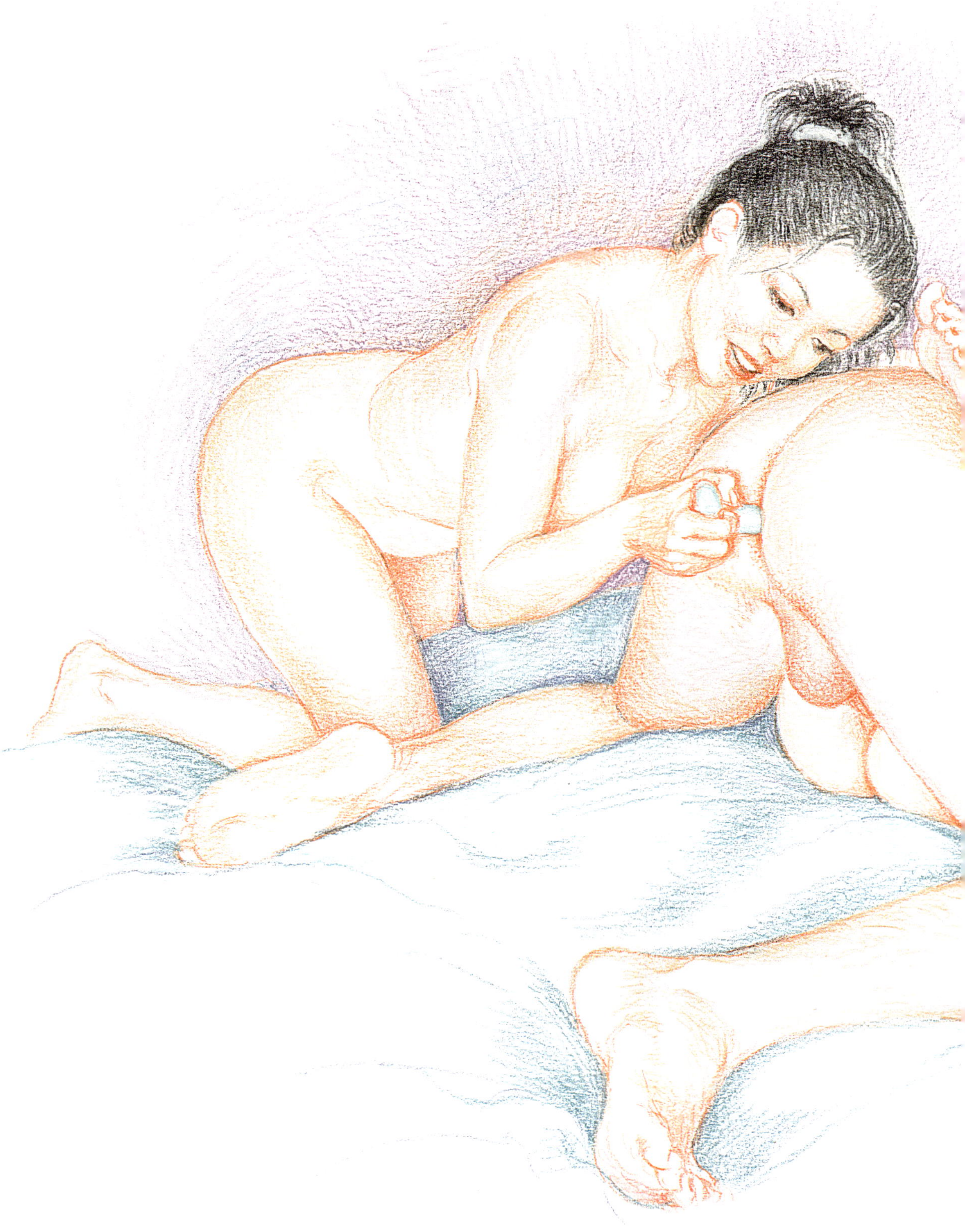

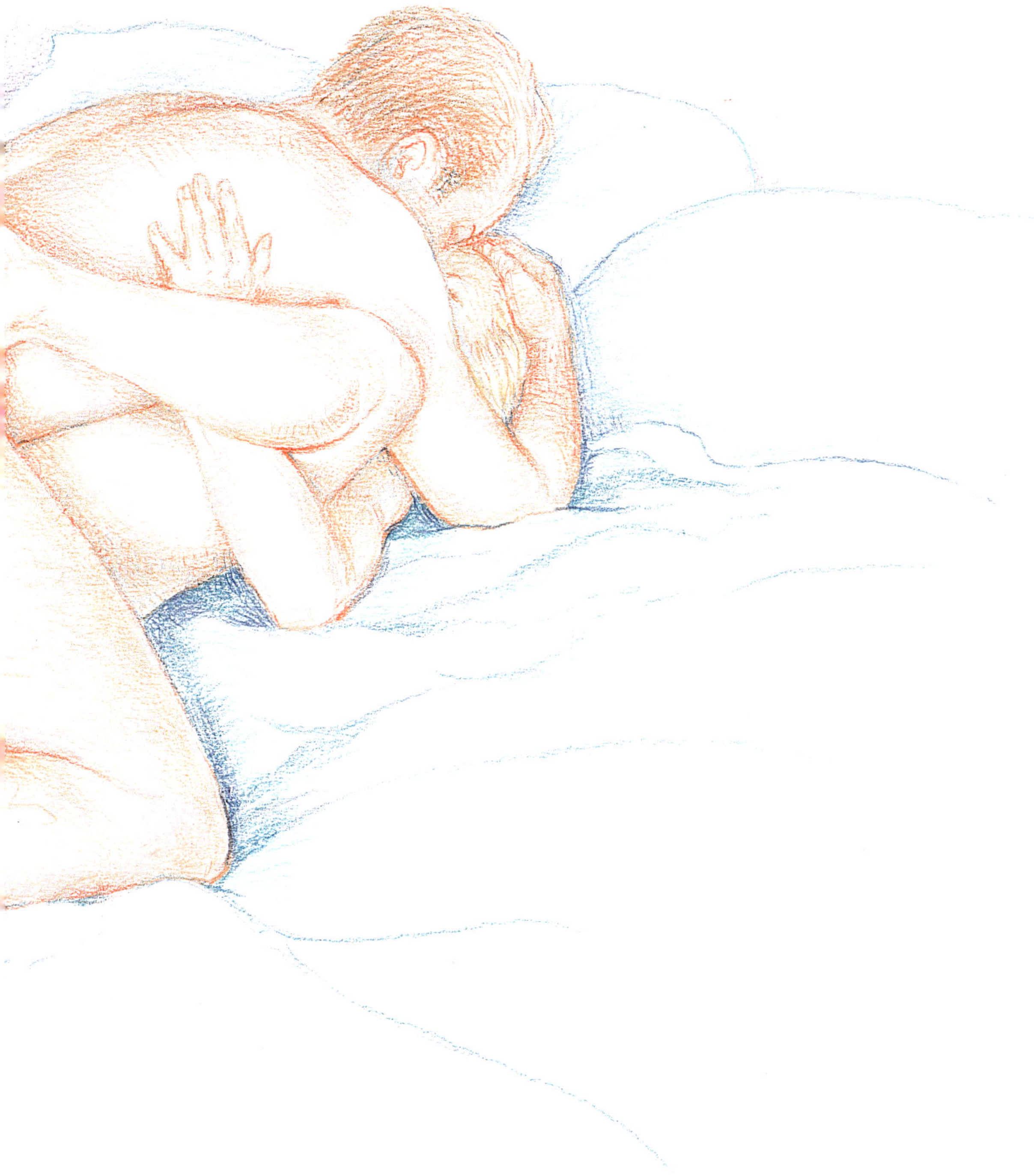

A Sensual Suprise

reading this will be quite envious of your relationship!

D This might at least make them realise that if they can only lighten up with each other, be sure that you love each other and have that depth of feeling; but you also are individual people.

P But for some people being jealous and possessive IS love! They think that is love when really it's nothing to do with love. It is about their own ego, and an image they have...

A I remember we had a meeting at work and there was a TV on in the background. There was one of these daytime chat shows on and it caught the attention of everyone in the room. They were all male. A man on the telly was saying, 'I'm quite happy seeing my wife being fucked by another man...'. I was sitting there saying nothing but everybody else in that room was so testosterone-driven; they were saying things like, 'If I ever saw my wife doing that I'd kill her!' They were all giving their reactions and all of them were negative, full of jealousy and selfishness...

D What did you say to them?

A I didn't say anything. It's not just other men being involved with their wives that worries some people: I remember having a long talk with a close friend of mine who needed a shoulder to cry on. We drank a whole bottle of liqueur together. He told me that he had come home and found his girlfriend, who is absolutely gorgeous, in bed with another girl. He walked into the room, and they said, 'Come and join us!' At this point I wondered

butterscotch sauce). If you've drawn the line at his penetrating your friend, you can straddle his erection, while she kneels over his face in order for him to lick her pussy.

If you bring along all those toys and strap-on dildos there is no end to the variations that can be created in threesomes. Adding one to two increases the possibilities immediately as well as heightening the energy and excitement. With experience, we start to develop a new sensitivity and helpfulness – if a cock slips out, you can help to put it back in again; if an extra tongue is needed, you can provide it.

For two women, if you haven't already tried it, the double dildo is a must (see illustration, next page). It may take a little time to get the hang of it but if your partner is there he will be delighted to lend a helping hand. The silicone variety is to be highly recommended.

Finding the ideal woman to join a threesome is not possible for everybody, for she must be just the right one for you and, hopefully, not sneaking off from her own husband, but equally not a lonely, frustrated single person who might get too emotionally caught up. If, by some stroke of fate, the right one does come along for you, enjoy it while it lasts for these relationships are often short-lived and intensely exciting. They should remain light-hearted and affectionate for if heavy emotion caused by possessiveness ever comes bubbling to the surface, the threesome is doomed.

Many couples who join the swinging scene find that once they have been to one or two events they will start to meet other couples naturally by a process of networking, so if your special woman has not put in an appearance yet, she may well turn up. You may form a friendship with a couple that later breaks up and one of them stays in contact; this is the way some threesomes happen.

Now we will return to our entertaining guide to look at another kind of threesome:

what the problem was! I couldn't believe it when he said that he had walked out. He told me that he couldn't abide the thought that he couldn't give her the pleasure that she wanted. He just kept asking, 'What does she want to go with another woman for?' I couldn't say anything to help; they finished the very next day. They had been living together and she had to pack her bags and go.

P I think a lot of these problems suddenly come up because people can't be honest with each other. Dishonesty is the most hurtful thing of all. There isn't that same sense of shock when you have been brought in and included. But on the other hand, I suppose we feel we have to conceal if our partner can't bear to hear the truth.

A I think that bisexuality is the biggest thing that people are dishonest about.

D Mm, guys as well.

P Do you think that men are more threatened by homosexuality than women are?

A Yes, they probably are. I would describe myself as bisexual.

D Well, yes, perhaps you are, but I have never known you crave a man.

P Bisexual women don't crave each other either, that's why it is more relaxed.

A You know I wouldn't have realised I could be bisexual until Debbie said that it would turn her on to see me with a man. We put an ad in to find a bi couple and

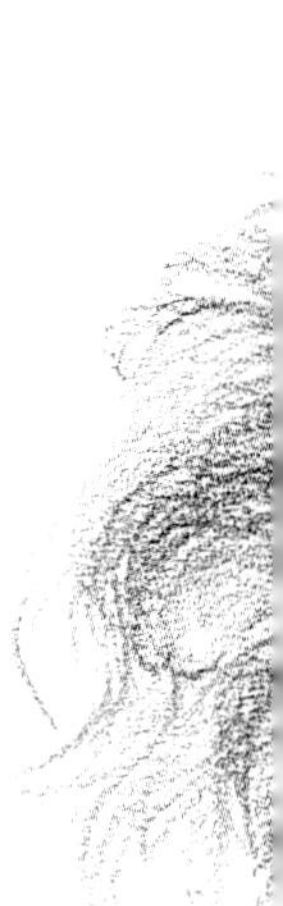

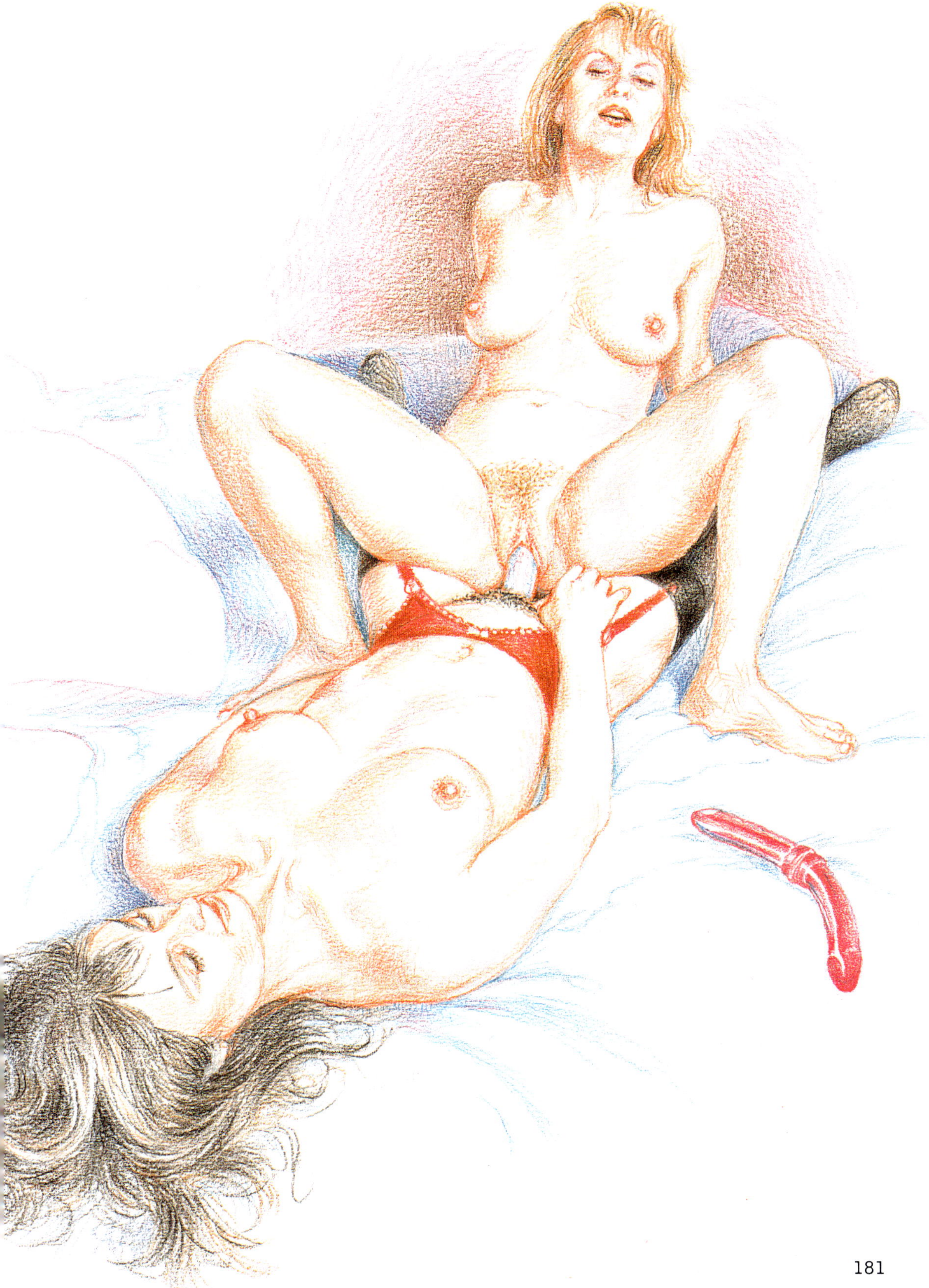

took it from there. It was all done in a very open way; we stayed in the same room together.

D I found it very exciting to watch the men playing together. I remember one time when the women played with each other... well, actually, she wasn't touching me, I was playing with her, but from where I was, I could see the two men, and that was a real turn on...

D ...but also, for you, if it never happened again with a guy it wouldn't bother you.

A No, not at all. I would never actually go looking for gay sex.

P The same thing must apply here as when a man is watching two women together. You get to see what men really like. I think we imagine gay men just getting straight down to it, and we still associate gentleness and foreplay with the feminine gender, don't we?

D Yes, women do need a lot of pre-attention. It doesn't all have to be gentle; once we are properly prepared we can be more responsive to the hard stuff!

A It was interesting that when we put in our ad looking for a bi man, we were absolutely inundated by replies, absolutely inundated, and 95% of those were from married men. They all said I'm bi but I can't tell my wife about it; she wouldn't accept it. It was quite an eye opener, because it makes you realise that there are a lot of bisexual men out there. I think that the vast majority of people are bisexual actually, but they haven't the courage to admit it.

D I think that a lot of people assume that anything to do with

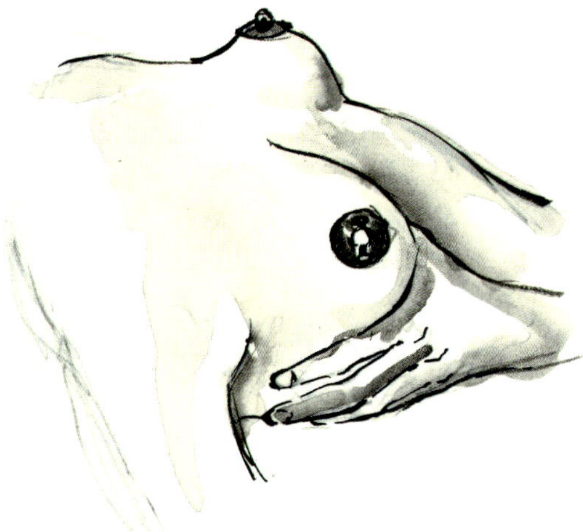

Having dealt with the scenario involving two women and a man, we now need to look at the other combination – one woman and two men.

Although I personally have had some wonderful times being the meat in a chap-sandwich, it is something I would hesitate to recommend to everyone without a word or two of warning; two sexually excited men is an awful lot of rampant testosterone for one girl to control. (Yes, I know the porn actresses make it look easy, but remember, they are very experienced, and so are the actors – and it's probably the third take, anyway.)

So, the most essential foreplay to this kind of threesome is – talk about it first. It helps to know what everyone's

gayness and men is going to include anal sex, but not all men want that. Sometimes it's just playing around and sucking... it's not like being gay as such, they are not having penetrative sex. So, I think that partners of bi men should just let them be themselves.

A The number of women we've met who've been turned on by it is phenomenal!

P Well, you've certainly gone a lot further than most people!

D Yes, I suppose we have, but you must remember we haven't done it all in one go. We've progressed over the years.

A The key is sharing and feeling that you are in control of what is happening. There has only been one instance where I felt unhappy when Debbie had arranged to meet up with a man on her own, but when we talked about it and she realised why I was upset we were able to sort it out. That's the main thing: if either of us is unhappy then we must be prepared to draw back and go no further.

D I completely agree. Being a couple together and making sure that everything is enjoyable for BOTH of us, is the most important thing.

expectations are before you start; do both men expect to have penetrative sex, or does one prefer to watch? Is one or are both guys bi? (This is very *important if one is, and the other isn't, and doesn't want to be.) If they both want to screw her, it's a good idea to establish a pecking order. This is also the time to establish the boundaries; the lady might not want full sex with the man who isn't her partner, in which case it's essential to get this straight before the panties hit the floor.*

Incidentally, I would strongly advise that at least one of the men should be a long-term partner whom the lady can trust to look out for her, who understands her reactions to stimuli, and who can be relied on to call a halt if she gets tired or distressed.

So, parameters established, how to get started?

A confident girl can settle the boys on the bed, turn on some sexy music and perform a striptease. Getting them to feel and stroke bits as they are gradually exposed, then dancing away to continue the strip is a super way to get all three of you turned on and ready to rock. For a woman there are few things more exciting than seeing a man who is becoming really aroused by your body and this way – you get it in stereo. Don't worry if you haven't got a size 10 body or a perfect sense of rhythm –

Swinging Experiences: Fiona and Wiliam

Paula Do you remember the circumstances that prompted you and William to consider the idea of swinging, or at least, opening up your sex life to include others?

Fiona We placed an advertisement in a contact magazine. That was twenty years ago. We didn't just do this out of the blue; there were incidents that led up to it.

P Before this new departure would you say you had a normal sort of marriage?

William Depends what you mean by normal. We had both been married before and both had had many, many partners. I myself had had what you would call an open marriage and I was used to it...

P Ah, so this wasn't a completely new departure?

F It certainly was for me. I had had other partners but a lot of my sex life had always been unsatisfactory, unfulfilling and I was always looking for something else. This was before I met William who started to open me up. But I was very disapproving because he had had a relationship with a woman before me who loved being beaten. She absolutely loved sex and loved William too and to make matters worse she was just living down the road from us! So when he told me that sometimes he used to take a strap to this woman, very much to her delight, I was absolutely horrified.

believe me, any man with a pulse is going to love it.

However, if you're not quite so confident, one of the best ways for a girl to feel in control of this kind of threesome is to assume a 'dom' role, and treat the blokes as sex slaves, ordering them to massage or stroke her, or to lick her pussy. As long as they are happy to play along, this can be a great way of relaxing into the more hardcore stuff, and a pair of men with any kind of sexual creativity and empathy can give a lady a really mind-blowing experience! (I remember the first threesome I had; one lovely man concentrated on licking my clitoris, while the other rimmed my anus. I thought I had died and gone to heaven.)

When she's ready (and ONLY then), she can turn her attention to the two very satisfying erections with which the gentlemen may now present her; depending on what was previously agreed, the sky is the limit. She can, for example, get the guys to lie side by side and have a choice of cocks to stroke, suck or ride; she can be penetrated on all fours by one man while taking the other in her mouth. This looks absolutely fantastic if you have a mirror anywhere near the bed, but the gentleman at the top end must pay particular attention to make sure she is breathing comfortably, as if she is supporting her weight on her hands, she might find it difficult to control how much penis is going into her mouth!

Of course, all porn videos love the 'double entry' shots, where the lady takes one man in her pussy, and the other in her anus. I hope it goes without saying that this should NOT be tried by either of the guys unless the lady has indicated her willingness, and of course, all the usual rules about anal sex (lubrication, preparation, hygiene) apply. Actually, this is surprisingly tricky to get right, and personally I'm not at all sure if the 'classic' position (lady rides man No 1, man No 2 penetrates her anus from behind) is the best. It always reminds me of those puzzles you used to get as a child, where you had to roll a number of ball bearings into little dents in a clown's face. As soon as you got the second one in, the first always slipped out…

You might find it easier to have the lady

P You were married at this stage?

F Well, we were living together and got married shortly afterwards. That was 27 years ago.

P So the relationship with the other woman finished then?

W Well, it sort of waxed and waned over the years… She was miffed that I had taken up with Fiona.

P How did your disapproval change into something else, Fiona? Were you willing to try new things?

F It all began with William discovering me on the phone with a lover. He was a young man I was working with and I had the hots for him, although it was more in the mind than the body – but that can be very disturbing. Anyway, there were lots of phone calls and William overheard one of them. So, that started the openness. He then told me about an affair he had been having and I can remember being so relieved. I was at last able to let go of all the guilt! Also, there was a new feeling of intimacy after being able to share those things honestly.

W Yes, and what happened next was that we had a threesome with this man! I don't remember precisely how it happened but it was very unsatisfactory – he was bloody useless!

P Did it just happen spontaneously?

W No, we talked about it first and decided it would be a good idea. Fiona said she would go along with

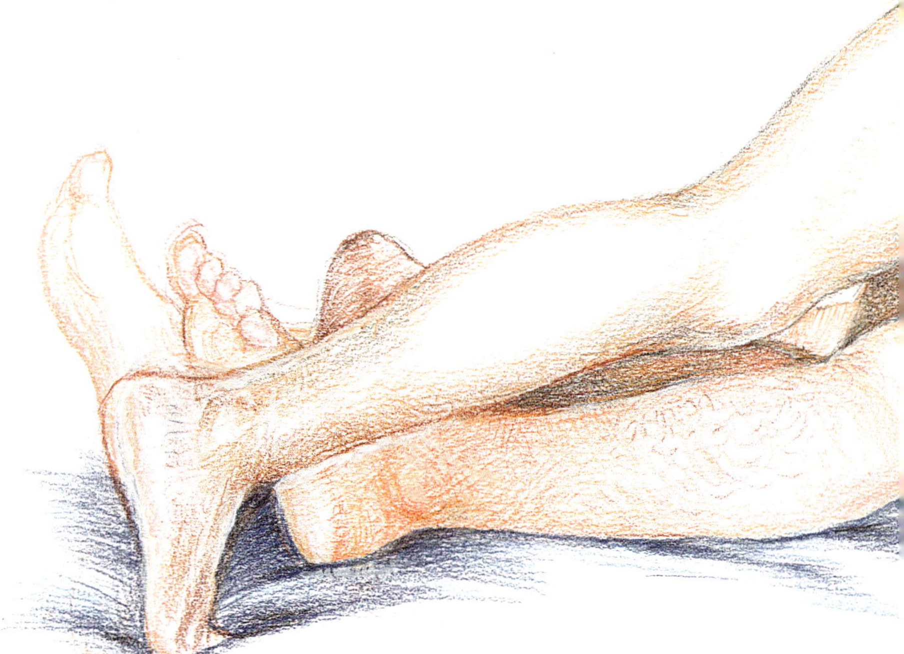

Double Penetration is quite
tricky to get right

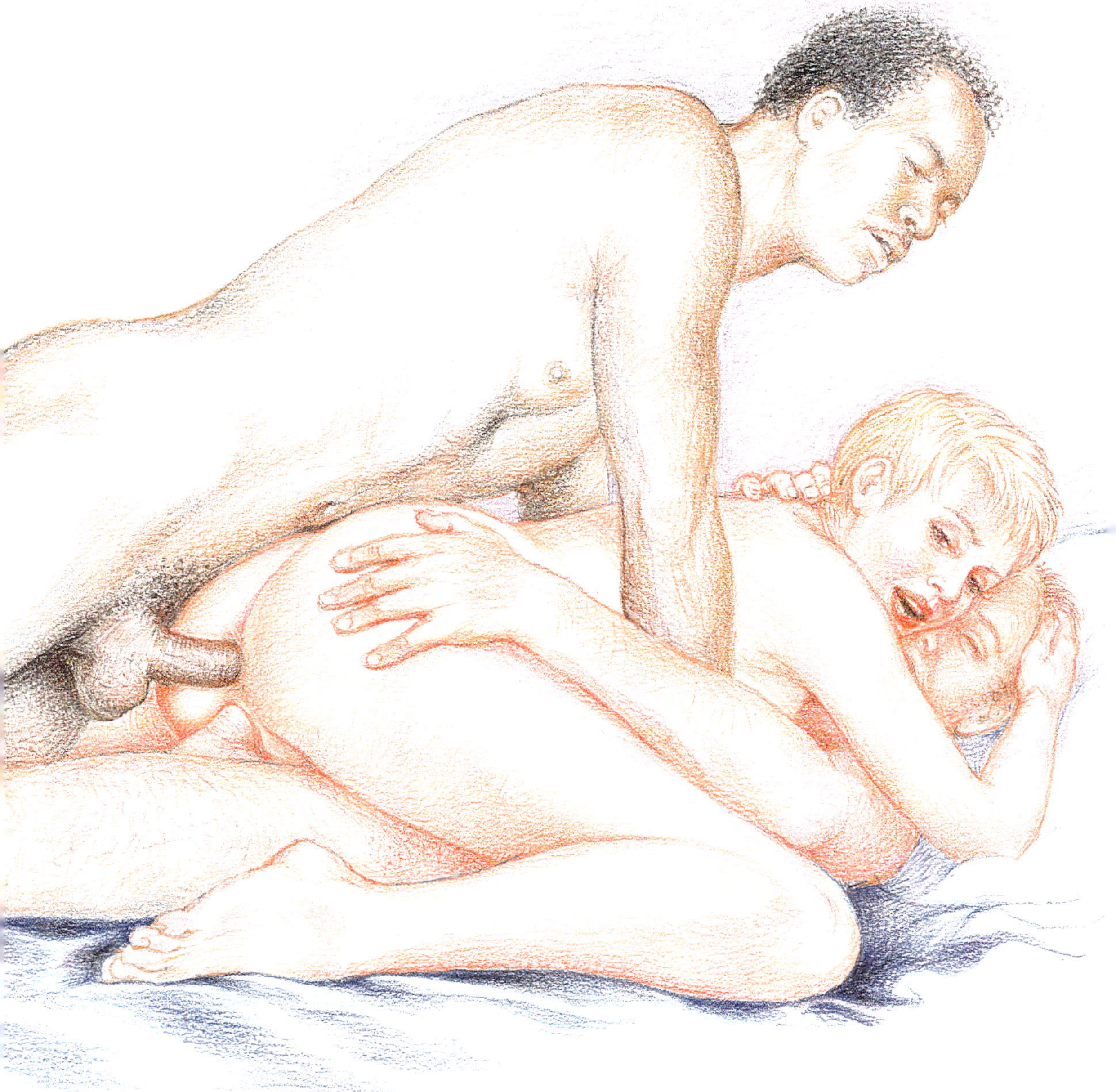

it. Anyway, although it was so unsatisfactory, it did set a tone...

F Oh yes, I remember now! I got very drunk...

P How did he react?

W He was very passive. I think he could have swung either way. I suspect he was bisexual, although he probably didn't really know himself. We knew at once that this relationship couldn't go anywhere... but that incident somehow opened up new possibilities. We talked a lot about it and then finally we decided we would advertise, to try to meet people who would be a bit more satisfactory. We put an advert in a contact magazine called 'Experience'. What was so amazing about this was that it was like suddenly becoming film stars – we just got masses and masses of mail. Letters from couples and singles and clubs and parties. It was endless. There weren't enough hours in the day to follow up all those invitations. It was all rather amazing.

Anyway, we chose a few, and met them somewhere first before we invited them to the house. We had a one night stand with a man who Fiona was very keen on, who just appeared out of the magazine and then disappeared again so that didn't lead anywhere. There were one or two like that but then we met a really wild couple who ran a pub and we were invited to a party they were organising. This was the breakthrough. We then started to network and it all took off.

P So the contact ad really worked for you?

lying on her side facing man No 1, with man No 2 lying facing her back; No 2 raises and supports her upper leg, thus facilitating No 1 entering her pussy. No 2 should then be able to access her anus fairly easily.

These are just a few ideas, and I'm sure you will have lots more fun finding your own combinations; just remember the importance of patience, awareness, and communication at all times – then just... enjoy it!

And before I forget – a word about booze. In a word, chaps – don't! Alcohol is no friend to the sexy threesome, as it dulls awareness, makes you morose and aggressive, and plays havoc with your ability to maintain an erection. Believe me, from a woman's point of view, one limp dick is depressing enough, but two is enough to put you off for life!

How will you both react to male bisexuality? Of course, threesomes can be thoroughly enjoyed without there being any emphasis on this aspect; two men can concentrate entirely on the woman they are pleasuring and not be troubled by each other's physical presence, but this is rarely the case for long and for a man it seems to be a more tricky issue to deal with. I know many women who feel entirely comfortable pleasuring each other; it is a beautiful and calming experience, a bit like turning away from the cut and thrust of a busy main road into a quieter country lane. For many men, however, the prospect of experimenting with homosexuality seems, understandably, to present a bigger threat to their self-image and security.

Heterosexual men can vary in their reactions. One friend told me that he could imagine enjoying being sodomised by another man because the sensations would be arousing, and he wouldn't have to look him in the face, but there was no way he could bear a man kissing him. Ugh! Yuck! I thought this a bit odd at first and then reflected that erotic kissing is probably the most intimate physical act of them all. I recall hearing a hard-working prostitute say, in an interview on TV, that she never did kissing with her clients – that

F ABSOLUTELY! It was the best ten pounds we have ever spent in our lives.

P But were there any unsuccessful contacts?

W Yes, there were – some. I should say roughly half and half. The famous, most unsuccessful one was this guy who had sent us a photo through the mail of this rather beautiful black man. We looked at it and thought, 'Mmm... we really like the look of HIM', and so we invited him directly to the house. This was the first time we had ever done this and it was a major mistake! The doorbell rang and there was this unattractive white guy. I said, 'You sent us someone else's photo,' and he replied, 'I thought you wouldn't invite me if I sent my own.' 'Too right,' I said. 'On your bike, sunshine!'

F We did have a few meetings with couples that didn't work out too well.

P Yes, that must be very awkward; when you are with a couple and say, William likes the girl but Fiona doesn't like the man at all.

W Yes, that can be very embarrassing. It's bound to happen though. I'm thinking of a couple from Southend. I thought she was alright but we both took against him in a big way. Then, what do you do with the evening? What do you say? I've known people feel rejected, get upset and then you have to deal with all that unnecessary emotion and that's not the name of the game. The name of the game is play and to have pleasure.

P Did you talk about your experiences afterwards?

W Oh yes! Endlessly, endlessly. In the beginning the new experiences were exciting and fulfilling, both sexually and for our fantasy life. After we came home from a successful 'do' we'd always have a really good bonk to finish it off...

F ...and there was so much discovery! Discovery AND excitement.

W Yes, pushing the boundaries and following the mind. Do you remember the writer Luke Reinhart? 'The Dice Man'? I know that's all sixties stuff, but it's that notion of following your mind. You make a decision that you're going to do something and then you follow it through and don't give in.

P You had that agreement between the two of you that you were going to follow through. But did you lay down any guidelines beforehand; were there any things you decided you were not going to do?

F There was a guideline we had from time to time which was that we would not go off into another room, but then there have been times when we've done exactly that! There have been times when I have said, very self-righteously, `I don't do solo,' and then I've gone off and had an affair!

W ... another thing is, we're not interested in being bi...

F But just lately I've become much more interested in it.

W Well, I've had a couple of bi

was reserved for her boyfriend only.

Everyone has different boundaries and we must try not to cross them, however unwittingly. Picture this scene; it happened at a sex party. A virile young man was lustily engaged in fucking his girlfriend (with him on top) while others offered encouraging caresses and gentle kisses to his back and bottom. Then a tongue began to snake between his buttock cheeks and I heard groans of pleasure coming from him. 'Oh yes, that's lovely,' he whispered, luxuriating in the sensation, 'more, more...' After a few minutes of this he looked round appreciatively and to his horror, realised that the tongue belonged to a man. That was the end! Not only was the young man appalled, he was so furious he could not continue. So let's be sensitive about this and not stir up any unwanted aggravation. Always make sure that you know where to draw the line before you start out.

FINDING A LIKE-MINDED COUPLE

Most couples start their search for swinging friends by advertising for another couple to join them. This seems the obvious leaping-off point, for you have got to start somewhere, but the more I hear about the results of these foursomes the more I feel that they are not the ideal set-up for a successful encounter.

I can remember the days when two couples meeting up for sexual pleasures was called 'wife swapping', which is a term liable to turn off any hot-blooded woman before she's even started. The idea implies that she is merely to be shunted from one male to the other, with little input from her along the way. The reality, of course, is that everyone has a very big input in the matter, and because of that there is rarely a case where each member of the foursome takes to the other with equal enthusiasm. You only need to think about it for a few minutes to realise that the likelihood of both members of one couple fancying both members of the

experiences, mainly in group situations where you're not quite sure who's got hold of your dick and you look down and see some geezer sucking it and you think, 'Oh, what's going on?'

P Did it make you feel 'Yuk'?

W No, it just made me smile! I suppose it's all part of the scene. It's not something I particularly want to do... But, getting back to what we were saying, it's very important, even though you don't necessarily keep to them, to have a discussion about having boundaries and guidelines. I've heard some couples say they have a secret word. You know, if one of them isn't liking what they are doing they say 'rhubarb' or something and then your partner can help you out. I think having discussions and setting guidelines help to make you feel safe.

F Yes, and as well as that there's always the feeling that whatever you do, you come back to base. And the other thing we talk about... we call it 'being in league'. It's as if we're in a secret, just the two of us, and we get pleasure from the fact that it is clandestine as far as our straight friends go. We don't want them to know because actually there's such a pleasure in the double life. SUCH fun.

W Of course, we can never really be sure that our friends aren't up to things too! But we'd rather keep the boundaries. With some of our close friends sex would be quite unthinkable. The interesting thing is though, that because of the particular group of people we got involved with, some of them have now become wonderful friends and because of that we don't have sex with them any more. I do think that's interesting – the transition, when a purely sexual relationship is translated into a friendship.

F I agree, when people are semi-strangers it's more exciting. That's because there's such an element of fantasy and discovery, and when you've gone down that path with someone, you reach a point where the relationship is either going to become a fully-fledged friendship or it is going to fizzle out because there isn't enough mutual interest to keep it going. In fact we were thinking just today, before we came to talk to you, that our life is so, so rich because of all this... and I would even say that, if it wasn't for this, we probably might not have stayed together. I think we might well have got bored, met other people and split up... or just drifted apart. And what is to me absolutely remarkable is that we now feel in our best phase sexually – the best we've ever been in! I would never have imagined that at the age of 58 I'd be having the time of my life. I think it's better than it was twenty years ago – very heightened, very exciting.

P Mmm... that just shows that you don't need excessive amounts of hormones to drive you – in fact, in a way they are responsible for making us go up and down. I remember feeling a sudden gush of desire and then that could easily swing into a different mood and I didn't feel like it any more. Nowadays my feelings are more constant and my mind is more in control.

F Yes, exactly. We've been

other is very remote. Then there is the unexpected possibility that the two women might suddenly develop a passion for each other and both of the men are left out in the cold. Anything can happen.

Great tact is needed when a meeting goes awry. There is nothing more offensive than being told that we are not fancied (it is highly embarrassing to have to tell someone that, too), and most of us who do not thrive on humiliation would rather avoid the occasion for it altogether. Spending time getting to know more about the potential partners seems a wise precaution.

Another helpful idea is to decide in advance what you are going to do if disaster strikes. Have some prearranged codewords to make it easier to communicate discreetly with each other and decide beforehand how you will politely extricate yourselves if it should be necessary. If you both choose to go ahead with the other couple, you also need to have agreed whether you are prepared to separate and go into different rooms with the new partner or remain in closer contact. To some this makes a big difference.

By far the best way to meet new, sexy, friends is at a well-organised swinging party. When there are several couples participating there is not that awkward pressure on each individual to join in whether they like it or not. If you happen to find yourself being bent back over the sofa by the most overbearing, sweaty-palmed individual in the room, it is much easier to excuse yourself at a party simply by saying that you need to refresh your glass. You then mince away blowing them a friendly kiss, and make sure you never come within a range of ten feet of them again. You just have to hope they will be hovering optimistically around someone else when you next set eyes upon them.

SWINGING PARTIES

When you have met a few amiable people and got on well in the early stages, you will sooner or later be invited to a party. Now we have arrived at the possible fulfilment of all your

through lots of ups and downs, especially when coming up to fifty.

W But we decided that we were both going to come through. And we did: we came through and found this strong relationship between us.

F Now we live our life completely in the present.

W You should never try to live in the past – or the future.

F We have had periods when we have withdrawn completely and I've thought, 'I'm never going to do that again.' It had all become meaningless. But I think that was because we had pushed through to yet another level of honesty.

W I think the time when we withdrew was during our children's difficult teen years. They really took every ounce of our energy at that time.

F And of course the occasional gynaecological problem does not help.

P Another question: do you think that men are likely to get more jealous and possessive than women, when they start to experiment with swinging?

F No, I don't. Women are much more likely to. On the whole they are allowed to do more by men, but I think they get much more jealous and threatened if their men wish to have the same freedom.

P That's unexpected! I have assumed that men were usually more possessive.

F That has never been my experience.

W Women have lots more opportunity to indulge themselves at parties. I can remember seeing a woman fucking with two men and having a whale of a time but the moment her husband got an erection and was obviously interested in another woman she went bananas!

P Perhaps women take it for granted – because of course they have more choice, don't they. They are often spoilt for attention, whereas men maybe have to work a little harder when they are at a party.

W But then of course the other side of that is the type of situation where it looks as though the woman is only there doing it all just to please the man; she doesn't really want to be there at all. You see that sometimes at the bigger parties.

P What about you two; has there ever been jealousy?

W Oh yes, of course..
F That's all part of it!
W The exquisiteness of the pain of jealousy is something quite particular.
F Not too much though... jealousy can destroy... but it can be a frisson.
W Yes, the right amount can be exciting... but we're aware of how it can destroy a marriage – we've seen it happen to friends of ours who are not in the swinging scene. One sexual infidelity and the green-eyed monster rears its ugly head... but I suppose that a relationship cannot be that strong if it caves in just because one of the partners has sex with someone else.

P Now can we talk about the S&M aspect of all this and whether

fantasies and daydreams! You have come this far, and want to enter the inner sanctum. Be prepared for some pretty heady experiences, but at the same time be aware that there is a form of etiquette that must be learned before you venture into a crowded room full of naked and semi-naked people.

Yes, all right; we're all gathered together here, just as worshippers congregate in a church, with more or less the same aim – the celebration of erotic love. but just because there is a common objective, it doesn't mean that everyone there just wants to get on with it with any and everybody. Sex doesn't work like that. It needs to be coaxed and tempted out with the same imagination and sensitivity needed in any ordinary, one-to-one seduction: this is just a speeded-up version.

You should never just concentrate on one person at a swinging party, for there is always their partner and yours to be considered and you need your antennae to be pointed in all directions to pick up what is going on and how everyone feels. That can be particularly difficult if you happen to have a throbbing hard-on, a state that tends to dictate some form of urgent action. But, you see, that's what this game is all about: apart from being a means to phenomenal sensual delights, believe it or not, swinging must also be a training and a discipline!

Are you prepared for the changes that may come about in you and your partner when you begin to release yourselves sexually? The differences could be particularly apparent in women who have been rather modest and passive in the past. Not all men are able to cope with this. They may be the ones who initially suggested a venture into this exciting new world and perhaps their partner only came along to be supportive, only to find herself caught up and completely swept away by an overwhelming rush of lust. The poor man looks on with horror as she pleasures herself with several hyperactive studs at once, with gasps, moans and orgasmic shrieks he has never heard before. He may see her emerge with a newly discovered potency

that started with just the two of you or is it something which only comes to life with other people?

W I'm just trying to think...no I don't think we've ever done it on our own...
F No, never in private.
W It never worked for us. I wasn't one for coming home on a Friday night and giving the missus a good walloping, but you do hear stories about couples that enjoy that sort of domestic arrangement!

P Yes, I get letters from readers of 'Februs' telling me about how their wife presents them with a list of her misdemeanours once a week and then she is taken upstairs for a good seeing-to.

W That sort of thing has never appealed to me. I've never been one for role-playing or games. Fiona has never dressed up as a maid for me, or anything like that. It has to be a direct relationship.

P You both strike me as being quite dominant people anyway.

W Yes, you've reminded me that used to be a really important issue that we talked about a lot. Fiona can be submissive, but it is only a performance...
F Yes, I'm definitely not a natural submissive but I do like the idea of some pain in sex... I love the idea of being smacked and pushed and shoved... and got at.

P Do you like it to be whole-hearted?

F Oh yes, I don't want to mess around.

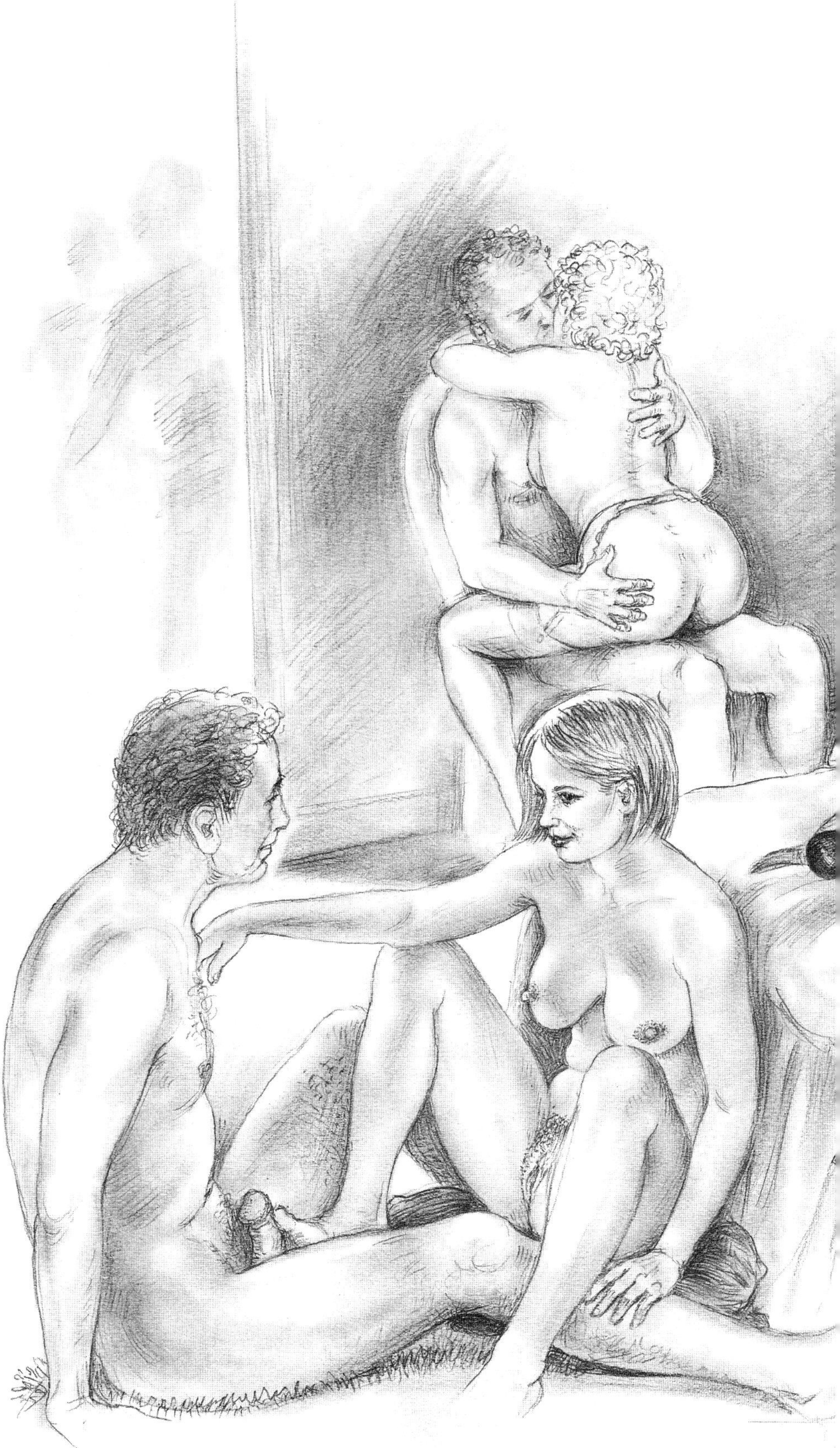

A Swinging Party

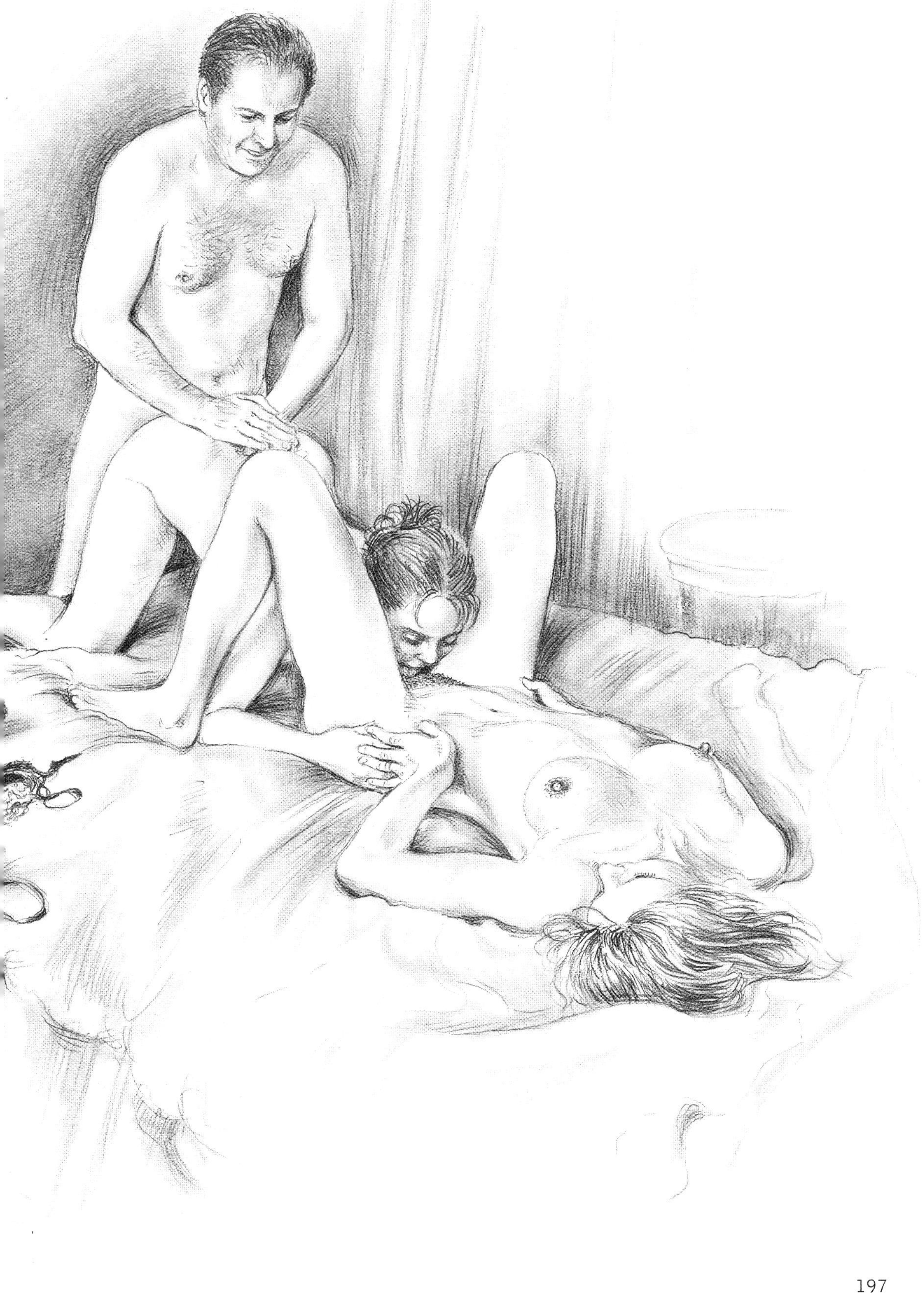

W But you like the show...
F Mm, yes, I love showing off!
W Remember when you were at the Club Doma... you took a very heavy whipping then.
F Yes, but I have no desire to be caned. I don't like that at all.

P There's never an element of punishment in any of the things you do...

W No, I wouldn't be interested in that. For me it has always been part of foreplay. When I've been whipping someone at a party or watched other couples engaged in sadomasochistic scenes, I find it's a direct route to intimacy and, in a way, almost a substitute for intimacy.

P It breaks down barriers.

W Yes, perhaps 'substitute' is the wrong word. Perhaps 'short cut' is better. With a submissive person I can get to be very intimate with them in a short period of time.

P Perhaps it's like a simulation – conjuring up an intimacy that isn't necessarily real.

W Exactly – unreal, perhaps, but more intense than the sort of normal sex party intimacy.

P Literally 'whipping something up'! Does holding a whip in your hand make you feel powerful or do you prefer spanking with your hand?

W Well, being a bit of a techno-anorak I have always loved beautifully made implements.

that will change the balance of their relationship in a radical way.

For a woman, discovering her fully awakened sexuality can give her enormous confidence and inner power. At last she knows that women control the reins of sex; they can ignite its flame and they can extinguish it; they can initiate it in their own way and do not have to wait for a man to make the first move.

Obviously, not all women will get the same benefits from swinging. Perhaps even more than men they can be thrown by a sudden stab of jealousy when another woman who may be younger, prettier and slimmer, starts to take an interest in their man, even when she has just indulged herself to the full and knows it is unfair to begrudge him an equal freedom. All these powerful emotions must be grappled with. Some find they can come to terms with it – and some cannot.

I believe that the most successful sex parties are always those where the women are permitted to take the lead.

There should be a good balance of couples. It is harder to make a party work if there are several unaccompanied men, for obvious reasons, although it never seems to bother anyone if there are several single women.

This is a world where women have the most astonishing advantages and can really come into their own. All you restless males out there who are on the brink of taking the plunge, you have been warned; if you don't wish to let that particular genie out of the bottle, then do not go down this path.

It also must be stressed that honesty is a necessity if swinging is going to be successful for you and your partner. Don't underestimate how difficult that can be. It is like being naked all the time. At first we're not used to it.

The last word on the subject must be about health for we cannot overestimate the importance of looking after ourselves – and others we come into contact with. Most parties will provide copious supplies of condoms, but always come prepared, and make sure you do not use the same one if you go

P And you are not averse to picking up a whip yourself – I can remember years ago watching you, Fiona, as you circled around a man who was tied to a pillar, teasing him with your riding crop. How your eyes flashed as you contemplated him! I think some spirit entered into you at that moment. I'll never forget that image – you looked like a goddess! Enjoying your power over him...

F Oh yes, I loved that!

P But you are never like that with William, are you?

F Oh no, never.

P Now I want to ask you about when things have gone wrong and you've had terrible rows, and what has caused the rows.

W We've had the most horrific rows on the way back from events – not often, maybe about six times in all – and they have usually been caused by the fact that Fiona has enjoyed herself much more than I have. It's not that I was moaning about it – just that she gets angry with me for not having a better time and then feels guilty about it.

P You said earlier that meeting up with a couple can lead to uncomfortable situations when one of you reacts favourably and the other does not. This seems to be a risky business.

W Oh yes, it can be. I remember one occasion when we met a new couple and I couldn't respond to the woman at all, whereas the man was hot for Fiona. She wasn't particularly bothered by him but being a trooper she did her business! But there was no way I could do anything with the wife – and that was that. On the way home Fiona was beside herself with rage...

P So, parties are better really aren't they? For meeting people... and if you don't want to go any further with someone you can drift off and get involved with others without causing too much offence.

W Hmm... yes, come to think of it we have never had a really successful meeting with a new couple from advertisements. There was only one, but we met them first at a party.

F Definitely, parties are the best place for meeting couples. If you meet people you like you can then make arrangements to meet again. Small groups are the best.

W We recently went to Paris for a long weekend and had a terrific time going to clubs. We went to three different clubs and had a wonderful time. They were so different from clubs we've experienced here: clean, spacious, with food and entertainment, sophisticated and civilised, rather than some hole-in-the-wall hotel in Camberwell. It's that whole misunderstanding of what sex is all about in British culture.

F I do think that the exploration and discovery and excitement has been very influenced, the quality of it, by the quality of the people we've met. We have very special long lasting friendships, and now when we get together, although I don't have the sexual feeling for them any more, there is a huge

from one lover to another. It is very easy in the heat of the moment to overlook all other considerations apart from the immediate satisfaction of your desires, but believe me, it is far better the next day to have peace of mind than to be worrying endlessly about whether you have caught an infection or might have spread one. I know disease is not a particularly sexy subject, but unfortunately it is a fact of life that can attack us at the very heart of our favourite pleasure. So take care, and play safely and wisely.

CLUBS

Visiting a swingers' club can be a revelation, if you are one of those who come alive amidst throngs of people. For most of us, the small, intimate gathering of sympathetic friends is more fulfilling, but on occasion the club atmosphere can provide exactly what we need, offering a wonderful opportunity to get into our most outrageous or flamboyant attire and let out the exhibitionist in ourselves. The only problem is that swinging clubs in this country are variable, both in the quality of the location and the way they are organised. You will hear all kinds of anecdotes about clubs, some recalling the most successful events where the people were friendly as well as horny and revelries reached sensual heights worthy of a Dionysian orgy. On the other hand, there are occasions when the atmosphere is all wrong and you know from the outset that nothing much is going to happen. One of my girlfriends told me how she and her husband had turned up at a new club that advertised a special 'hungry girls night'. As they looked around they realised that more and more men were turning up and standing around expectantly. Then one other woman appeared with her husband and my friend had the shocking realisation that the two of them were supposed to be the entertainment for the entire masculine horde! As it happened, both women took to each other and decided they would try to salvage the evening as best they could. They chose two men each (apart from their husbands) and

warmth and also... appreciation, to know people like this. We have an intimacy based on shared experiences.

W We were thinking back to when I was at school, when I was about thirteen, and I was talking about sex with a friend of mine, as we did endlessly in those days. I was masturbating to images that were not very well formed – I hadn't read books like 'The Story of O' yet (that was a real watershed for me). Anyway, I was talking to this lad at school and – it has always stuck in my mind – he said, 'But is that REALLY all there is? Isn't there anything more than just... fucking? That sounds very boring.' To think, there you are aged thirteen with the whole of life before you, you've reached this foothill and you think, 'There MUST be something else!'

F And of course there is... LOTS more... If you were condemned to the missionary position, or any other position for the rest of your life you would certainly go off sex. You simply wouldn't bother.

W And yet we know people who seem to be happy with the perfunctory approach. If that's what sex means to them – then fine, but it certainly wouldn't suit us. Heightened eroticism, that's what it's all about...

F Yes, heightened eroticism! And after all this time, we're still learning new things about each other. We never STOP learning. As a woman, I am so pleased that I dared to take a risk and didn't just remain passive. Dare to do, and ask, and say... and the rewards will be great!

sent the rest of them packing, then choreographed the whole scene to suit themselves.

There is no doubt that the best clubs are in Europe, particularly France. These clubs reflect a totally different, more sophisticated approach towards the swinging life-style where proper attention is paid to etiquette, mixed in with pleasant surroundings and good food. When you are in Paris, a useful little guide to buy is 'Paris Sexy'. This will give you all the information you will need for a thoroughly stimulating weekend.

If you are an Internet user, you should have no trouble accessing the websites for swingers around the country and these will let you know what is happening near you.

For those who feel more fascinated by the fetish scene there are helpful websites, chat rooms and activities galore. This is now a very highly developed social network. For those of you who have never been to a fetish club, here is another quote from Grace Lau's book. She provides a memorable picture of her first foray into a London fetish club to find models for her photographs:

What first struck me in the dim underground club was the vision of pure theatrical presentation in fantastical costumes. Silently slinking through the dense, heavily-expectant atmosphere, or suggestively swaying to the metal music beat, there moved 'aliens' from the future adorned in studded leather cat suits and harnesses; clinging rubber corsets; thigh boots with 5-inch stiletto heels; shiny PVC, chain mail, masks and hoods; and plenty, plenty of bare unashamed flesh. Flaunting flesh that sweated and wobbled and that bore red raw signs of abuse, abuse by whip and cane or one of the many punishment-toys that were being conspicuously wielded, mainly by women.

If you want to go to one of these clubs you will usually be required to wear the appropriate attire and enter into the spirit of the evening; these are not places for uninvolved spectators.

DO MEN AND WOMEN HAVE DIFFERENT ATTITUDES AND NEEDS?

When I first considered this question I thought I had the answers all clear but the more I thought of the real people I actually knew, the more exceptions to my generalisations seemed to present themselves.

Let's consider some of the things often said by women about their attitudes to sex. It is commonly held that females are, in the main, only interested in sex when it is connected to love and relationships and therefore will not be as interested as men in encounters that involve sex purely for its own sake. Now this may be what women believe about themselves but it isn't necessarily true. Women are certainly more interested than men in meaning and context for an erotic encounter so that their first concern when meeting a new man would be, 'Will I like him?' rather than, 'Is he well hung?' Men are much more likely to be fixated on the physical details – what they are actually going to do, and whether the new woman has a nice body.

On the whole, though, I have found that there are similar percentages of both men and women who like one-night stands and 'zipless fucks'. Most of them choose this pattern of unemotional 'shagging' because they haven't been awakened romantically yet. The couples that choose to go into swinging are different, because usually they have found their partner and wish to extend their horizons, with the partner as the central emotional security. From this position of security both men and women can begin to really enjoy pure sex with renewed pleasure, adding skill, sensitivity and imagination, seasoned with emotional control and a degree of affection for all the fellow explorers with whom they come into contact.

This question may have been answered differently in the years before reliable contraception, for then of course women's attitudes would have been different, for reasons too obvious to go into.

Perhaps there are biological reasons for men's apparent ability to have affairs more readily than women; the fact remains that they find it easier to keep their extramarital exploits separate from their home life than women do. This could be because they have had centuries of practice, where worldly pursuits required constant separation from wife and family.

The distinction between one sort of sexual nature and another is much more clearly seen if we forget the division of the genders and define people more by whether they use sex for love or for power. I have met members of both genders who have oriented their sex drive completely to serve power. They will use their own erotic talents to get what they want, as well as manipulate others, and never give themselves unless there is something in it for them. Power is the big aphrodisiac and guides their choices. Those who worship at the other shrine will be the types who can only give for the love of giving and they may, like the Marquis de Sade's hapless 'Justine', be vulnerable to exploitation by others.

In reality, we have probably all had our feet in both these camps from time to time in our lives. All the same, I personally believe that although building your own power and learning how to wield it is a vital part of development for all of us, sex, as a drive, is much better off when safely placed in the love category. Without that ingredient it has a tendency to become hollow and meaningless.

One of the main purposes of sex is to be life affirming and joyous – all the more reason to use it for cherishing one another. The moment sex loses that essential flame perhaps it's time to take a break and reflect for a while. This is a journey of discovery and each explorer will find something unique.

appendix i

Couple-Friendly Sex Shops

Harmony
167 Charing Cross Road
London
WC2H 0EN
Web: www.harmonyxxx.com
Email: sales@harmonyxxx.com

Sh! Women's Erotic Emporium
39 Coronet Street
Islington
London
N1 6HD
Tel: 020 7613 5458
Fax: 020 7613 0020
Web: www.sh-womenstore.com
Email: sh@sh-womenstore.com

Agent Provocateur
6 Broadwick Street
London
W1V 1FH
Tel: 020 7439 0229
Web: www.agentprovocateur.com
Email: info@femmeboudoir.com

Paradiso
41, Old Compton St
London
W1D 6HJ
Tel: 020 7287 2487
(retail outlet for PVC clothesmakers with four way stretch)

Coco de Mer
23 Monmouth Street
Covent Garden
WC2
Tel: 020 7836 8882
Web: coco-de-mer.co.uk
Email: info@coco-de-mer.co.uk

While The Erotic Print Society may recommend retailers throughout this book based on our own happy experience of them, we will not and cannot be responsible for any transactions or communications between any third party and our readers.

Femme Boudoir Sensual Fashions for Women
17b Riding House Street
London
W1W 7DT

Tel: 020 7637 5794
Fax: 020 7637 5796
Web: www.femmeboudoir.com
Email: info@femmeboudoir.com

Ann Summers
In almost every major city in the UK

Tel Customer Care: 01883 629 320
Web: www.annsummers.com

Myla
Selfridges
Oxford Street
London
W1A 1AB

Tel: 08717 170515.
Web: www.myla.com
Email: services@myla.com

Gash
19 Westfield Terrace
Devonshire Quarter
Sheffield
S1 4GH

Tel: 0114 276 3733
Fax: 0114 273 9793
Web: www.gash.co.uk
Email: info@gash.co.uk

Useful Websites

www.blissbox.com
Erotic toys, gadgets and videos

www.davidspain.com
Erotic metal corsetry

www.dirty-david.com
Swingers Website

www.xandria.com
American based sex toys retailer

www.medicaltoys.com/dungeonbox.htm
Dungeons in a box

www.dungeon-enterprises.com
Dungeon and bondage equipment

www.loveisdivine.co.uk
Fetish Fashion Mail Order Company

www.british-naturism.org.uk
British Naturism Website

www.informedconsent.com
Fetish contact site

Magazines and Publications

The Erotic Review
A literary read for lovers of sophisticated erotica
Subscriptions Contact: 01732 744 038
www.TheEroticReview.co.uk

Desire Magazine
Moondance Media
The only erotic magazine for both women and men.
Contact : 020 7820 8844
Web: www.desire.co.uk

Forum Magazine
Northern and Shell
A letters and stories magazine, also good for contacts.
Subcriptions Contact: 01772 833 053

Skin Two
Fetish Magazine
Subscriptions Contact: 020 7498 5533
Web: www.skintwo.com

Janus & Februs
Spanking Magazines
See Janus Shop details

Bibliography

Sex Play
By Dr. David Delvin
The Erotic Print Society
ISBN: 189899840X
Contact: 0800 026 25 24

The Illustrated Book of Sex Gadgets
By Vicky and Charlie
The Erotic Print Society
ISBN: 1898998299
Contact: 0800 026 25 24

The Seductive Art of Japanese Bondage
By Midori
Greenery Press
ISBN: 1890159387

Adults in Wonderland
By Grace Lau
Serpents Tail
ISBN: 1852425520

Paris Sexy 2002 - 2003
By Yves Le Monnier
La Musardine
ISBN: 2842711637

The Ultimate Guide to Anal Sex for Women
By Tristan Taomino
Cleis Press
ISBN: 1573440280

The Essential Guide to the Practices of Corporal Punishment
By Lucy Bailey
Miss Marchmont's English Spanking Society
www.missmarchmont.com

A Hand in the Bush: The Delicate Art of Vaginal Fisting
By Deborah Addington
Greenery Press
ISBN: 1890159026

Other Useful Addresses

The Janus Bookshop
40, Old Compton Street
London
W1V 5PB
Tel: 020 7439 4389
www.januslondon.co.uk

Rigby & Peller
2, Hans Rd
Knightsbridge
London
SW3 1RX
Tel: 020 7589 9293
Web: www.rigbyandpeller.com
(Corset and Lingerie Retailers)

Alex Jacob (Whipmaker)
BCM Cobra
London
WC1N 3XX
Tel: 020 8316 2349
Fax: 020 7619 9444
Web: www.cobrawhips.com
Email: Alex@cobrawhips.com

INDEX

A

B

C

D

E

F

G

H

I

J

K